Breast Cancer

Breast Cancer

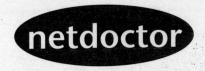

Series Editor
Dr Dan Rutherford
www.netdoctor.co.uk

Hodder & Stoughton
LONDON SYDNEY AUCKLAND

The material in this book is in no way intended to replace professional medical care or attention by a qualified practitioner. The materials in this book cannot and should not be used as a basis for diagnosis or choice of treatment.

Copyright © 2003 by NetDoctor.co.uk
Illustrations copyright © 2003 by Amanda Williams

First published in Great Britain in 2003

The right of NetDoctor.co.uk to be identified as the Author of the Work has been asserted by them in accordance with the Copyright, Designs and Patents Act 1988.

10 9 8 7 6 5 4 3 2 1

British Library Cataloguing in Publication Data
A record for this book is available from the British Library

ISBN 0 340 86141 X

Typeset in Garamond by Avon DataSet Ltd,
Bidford-on-Avon, Warwickshire

Printed and bound in Great Britain by
Bookmarque Ltd, Croydon, Surrey

The paper and board used in this paperback are natural recyclable products made from wood grown in sustainable forests. The manufacturing processes conform to the environmental regulations of the country of origin.

Hodder & Stoughton
A Division of Hodder Headline Ltd
338 Euston Road
London NW1 3BH
www.madaboutbooks.com

Contents

Foreword

Breast cancer is increasingly common. However, breast cancer is a complex problem, with ongoing scientific research and clinical trials continuing to make progress in our understanding of the cancer. Our knowledge of the disease and the way health professionals talk about it to patients can be confusing.

This book provides an approachable explanation to some of the causes and how we diagnose it, investigate and then treat breast cancer. It presents an overview which should be useful to friends and family as well as patients (both men and women) with breast cancer.

Whether you are facing breast cancer for the first time or whether you have known about the disease and how it affects people for a while, I hope you will use this book as the starting point to find out more.

Alastair M. Thompson
Professor of Surgical Oncology and Honorary Consultant Surgeon
University of Dundee

Acknowledgements

This book would not have been possible without the help provided by several people. In particular I thank Professor Alastair M. Thompson, Professor of Surgical Oncology and Honorary Consultant Surgeon at the Department of Surgery and Molecular Oncology, University of Dundee, who reviewed the text in detail despite a very busy workload and made many helpful suggestions and corrections.

The goal of this book is to provide an account of breast cancer that is sufficiently detailed to be useful while remaining understandable by the lay reader. Gail Davidson very kindly reviewed the book from the patient's perspective and encouraged us to feel that we were on the right track. I thank her sincerely for taking the time to do so.

The team at Hodder are always due thanks: Julie Hatherall, Sarah Grant, Patrick Knowles and Judith Longman in particular, and Amanda Williams for her artistic skills. My home team of Anne and David keep me right in every other respect.

Great care is taken in the production of the NetDoctor book series to ensure that the information is accurate, but if there are any errors then the responsibility is mine. Please let me know if you spot any. Suggestions for improvement in the content of the books are also welcome. Please send any comments to me at d.rutherford@netdoctor.co.uk

Dr Dan Rutherford
Medical Director
www.netdoctor.co.uk

Chapter 1

About the Breasts

Introduction

Breast cancer arises in a million women around the world every year, making it one of the commonest female cancers. For reasons that are not yet well understood it is a disease that is more common among 'Western' populations; rates of breast cancer in Far Eastern countries are about a fifth of those in the West. Breast cancer is commonest in older women and the proportion of older people in different countries is not the same, but once statistical adjustments are made for this so that countries can be compared with each other, the UK achieves the unenviable position of having the highest rate of breast cancer in the world, and that rate is climbing.

Breast cancer realities

As bare facts the figures may sound quite alarming; in the UK each year 39,000 women are diagnosed with breast cancer. Yet in absolute terms breast cancer is not a very common disease. Out of every thousand women at the age of 50, breast cancer will have arisen in only 20, or 2 per cent. The average life span of a woman in Britain now is very nearly 80 years, at which age about 3.5 per cent of women develop breast cancer each year. The lifetime risk of developing breast cancer is 1 in 11. Most British women therefore live long lives unaffected by breast, or any other, cancer.

In theory then, breast cancer should not be seen as a disease that lies in waiting for every woman as, statistically, it is not likely to happen. Statistics are of course all very well, but the reality of breast cancer to the individual woman is what matters. Breast cancer is a feared illness, and a diagnosis of breast cancer can have a dramatic impact upon a woman and her family. There is the fear of dying, because we tend to think of all cancers as fatal conditions, yet over 75 per cent of women with early breast cancer are still alive five years after diagnosis. There is the fear of coping with the loss of a breast, although mastectomy is by no means inevitable in the treatment of the disease and the results of breast conserving or reconstructive surgery are now excellent. There is the fear of radiation treatment, drug treatments (such as hormones and anti-cancer drugs) and their side effects, yet most such treatments are now very well tolerated. So even when breast cancer is no longer a statistic but is a personal fact the odds are strongly in favour of surviving for a long period of time. It's true that in a small proportion of women with breast cancer, particularly some of those affected at a young age (under 40 years), the course of the illness can be aggressive and rapidly fatal. One can't and shouldn't try to minimise the devastating effect it can have in those circumstances. But for the vast majority of women who develop breast cancer it is important to realise that it is a treatable illness that is perfectly compatible with an excellent quality and length of life thereafter.

Knowledge helps

It's entirely natural for us to feel anxious when we are unwell, but knowledge of what it is that's wrong, and what to expect along the way to recovery, greatly lightens the burden of illness. Even when cure is not possible it's good to know that there is treatment available.

This book summarises present knowledge about breast cancer in a form suitable for the non-medical reader, but it does not attempt to simplify information at the expense of accuracy. It avoids unnecessary jargon, but includes and explains technical terms when required. Breast cancer is an intensely active field of scientific and medical research and knowledge is changing. Some of the concepts we now believe to be accurate will undoubtedly change in the future – perhaps even the near future. We see this happening in almost every area of medicine, partly as a consequence of our expanding grasp of the fundamental processes of biology and of the genetic background to illness. All cancers are basically cells that have escaped the normally strict regulation governing their behaviour. We know much more than we did just a few years ago about what mechanisms keep healthy cells in order and what are the important influences that can break this control.

We're well justified in being positive about breast cancer, but there are many areas of controversy. We don't fully understand what causes any type of cancer, there are differences of opinion on what the best treatments are and how best to use them and there are many treatments under study (in clinical trials) about which we're still gathering the necessary information. But good treatments are available right now, and we have the expertise in the UK to benefit from them as much as, or better than, anywhere else in the world.

The logical place to start in understanding breast cancer is with a description of the structure and function of the breast.

Structure of the breast

Prior to puberty the tissues of the breast are exactly the same in females and males. At puberty the ovaries in a girl begin to produce increasing amounts of the female sex hormones, oestrogen and progesterone, and these have pronounced effects upon the growth and development of breast tissues. (A small amount of growth of breast tissue is often seen in teenage boys, again due to the changes in the sex hormones in boys of this age. This usually settles and fades away without treatment.)

The basic structure of the female breast is illustrated in figure 1. Within each breast there are about 20 groups (called lobes) of milk-producing glands, each one of which is called a lobule. Each lobule has a small tube leading from it, called a ductule, and these ductules link up to eventually form a wider tube (duct) that ultimately opens on the surface of the nipple. There are therefore about 20 of these duct openings on the nipple. The areola is the darker skin surrounding the nipple and the little lumps that are normally present on the areola (which are called Montgomery's tubercles) are not part of the milk duct system. When a baby is sucking at the breast it draws the nipple and the ducts under it well into its mouth and the rhythmic squeezing action of its mouth and gums draws milk in from each of the lobes.

The lobes are not rigidly distinct from each other in the same way as the segments of an orange but each lobe is a separate milk-producing zone. You can see this if an infection develops in a lobe, as it does sometimes in breastfeeding. Then a build up of inflammation and

Figure 1: Basic breast structure

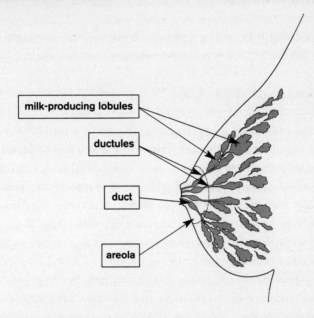

milk-producing lobules

ductules

duct

areola

pus can form but it is usually localised to one area of the breast, representing the infected lobe, and does not spread through the whole breast. In between the milk-producing lobules there is mixed a variable amount of fatty tissue plus the tough supporting tissues that maintain the shape of the breasts and which are linked to the muscles of the chest wall underneath. There is no muscle or bone within the breasts.

In most of a woman's life the breasts are not in milk-producing mode but even so it is not unusual for there to be some fluid discharge from the nipples from time to time. The exact nature and colour of this can vary enormously, although advice should always be sought if the discharge appears to be bloodstained. Most of the time that a nipple discharge occurs it will not be as a result of any serious underlying cause.

Lymph drainage

It's well worth knowing a bit about the system of lymph drainage from the breast, as it is very relevant to several aspects of breast cancer.

Lymph is a protein-rich clear fluid, present in virtually every part of the body, that mingles between the cells and effectively bathes all the tissues. Lymph is produced largely as the result of the effect of filtration of the blood through the tiny 'pores' in the smallest of blood vessels, the capillaries. These pores are too small to let through the red blood cells, which carry oxygen and give blood its red colour, hence lymph is almost colourless. Through the widespread network of tiny lymph-conducting tubes that eventually link up and empty back into the main veins, lymph is ultimately returned to the blood, so there is a continuous circulation of lymph to the tune of 2 or 3 litres per day in total. Normally this happens completely without fuss and we only become aware of lymph when for one reason or another its circulation becomes impaired. This causes lymph to accumulate in the tissues that are not being adequately drained, and these tissues then swell up.

A common example is the ankle and foot swelling that can accompany prolonged immobility in a sitting position, such as a long car or bus journey or a flight. Normally the pumping action of the calf muscles that happens when we walk about helps propel lymph back up the legs and onward into the main lymph drainage system. Sitting for prolonged periods stops this 'muscle pump' action, which has the knock-on effect of causing puffy ankles.

The flow of lymph through the lymphatic tube system is a one-way process, just as blood flows one way from the heart, through the arteries to the veins and then back to the heart. Each part of the body has its own 'lymph drainage' and, as human beings are built to a roughly similar design plan, so the lymph drainage of each part of

Figure 2: Lymph drainage of the breast, and lymph nodes

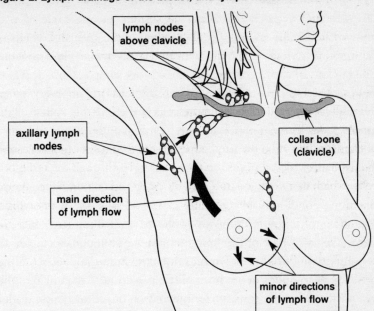

the body is well known. In the case of the breasts the drainage follows the pattern shown in figure 2, in which the majority (about 95 per cent) of the lymph drains to lymph channels located in the armpit. The medical term for the armpit is the axilla, so these are properly known as the axillary lymph vessels. A small proportion of the lymph drainage of the breast goes to channels running in the direction of the breastbone and towards the abdomen.

Lymph nodes

You'll notice that in figure 2 numerous small swellings are drawn along the lines of the lymph channels. These are known as lymph nodes and they are a feature of the lymphatic system throughout the body. Lymph nodes receive lymph, which passes through the node and out through exit channels that lead on to other lymph nodes 'downstream' in the lymph drainage system. Lymph nodes act as sophisticated filters and they contain many of the specialised cells of the immune system, which are activated if the lymph fluid contains foreign material such as bacteria or viruses for example. Once activated these sentry cells can send chemical messages via the lymphatic system and the bloodstream to recruit more cells of the immune system. Thus lymph nodes form an important part of the monitoring and response mechanism that protects us against infection and, as we'll see later, against cancer too.

You can in effect see the lymph nodes in action in common infectious conditions like tonsillitis. The tonsils are walnut-sized collections of tissue at the sides of the back of the throat (and are themselves also part of the immune system, although not made of the same type of tissue as lymph nodes). Lymph drainage from the tonsils goes to nodes in the front of the neck, under the angle of the jaw. In tonsillitis the tonsils are infected so the local lymph nodes swing into action, becoming swollen and tender. These swollen 'glands' are usually easily felt and as the tonsillitis recedes so the lymph nodes shrink back to their normal size, which is usually too small to be felt.

The axillary nodes are also sufficiently near to the surface of the skin to be felt when they are swollen, as are the lymph nodes in the groin. The axillary nodes also receive lymph from the whole of the arm and the groin nodes from the whole of the leg and foot, so when searching for the cause of swollen lymph nodes in these sites a doctor checks for signs of infection (the commonest cause of swollen nodes) on the whole of the limb. It's quite easy for an infected finger, for example, to be the reason for swollen nodes in the armpit on the same side.

Swelling of lymph nodes always needs an explanation. Most of the time nodes swell up over a short period of time in just one region of the body, are related to an obvious local infection and over a period of two or three weeks they become impalpable again as the infection is resolved. There are many other possible causes of lymph node swelling, including diseases of the immune system itself, in which nodes are more swollen than is usual for infection, in which the swelling affects many groups of nodes rather than just one and in which node swelling persists over many weeks or months rather than the short-lived pattern of simple infection. As with any new, unusual or persistent lump that you find on your body you should always report it to your doctor without delay and not just keep your fingers crossed that it will go away.

In relation to breast cancer, however, our interest in lymph nodes is that one of the several ways in which all cancers spread to other parts of the body is via the lymphatic system. As we'll see later in more detail, part of the process of examining a woman with breast cancer involves determining whether the cancer has moved from its origin in the breast to one or more of the lymph nodes that drain the breast. Such spread has important consequences for the type of treatment needed and, ultimately, on the survivability of the cancer. A woman with no spread of her breast cancer to the axillary nodes at the time of diagnosis has a greater than 80 per cent chance of being alive five years later. A woman with more than 10 lymph nodes involved at diagnosis has a less than 30 per cent chance of surviving this length of time.

Cancer in general

Breast cancer is but one of hundreds of different types of cancer that can arise from the many different types of tissue that make up the body. There are, however, certain general principles that apply to all cancers that we can use in trying to understand what cancer is, and why it has the effects that we see.

CELL STRUCTURE

The basic unit of living tissue is the cell. The simplest organisms, such as the amoeba, are made of single cells, whereas a human being has billions of cells. Although in complex beings like us our cells are divided into many different types capable of completely different functions they all have a similar general structure. They have an outer wall, or cell membrane, that controls the flow in and out of substances such as nutrients and salts. The cell membrane may also be sensitive to certain circulating trigger substances called hormones that have further actions within the cell. Inside the cell there is a fluid called cytoplasm, within which there are other structures that, for example, provide the cell with energy or which are engaged in the duplication process that allows cells to make exact copies of themselves. Most cells also have a nucleus, which contains the genetic code material, DNA, which is organised into tightly packed bundles called chromosomes. Human beings have 23 pairs of chromosomes, half of each pair coming from each parent.

A gene is a short section of this DNA code on a particular chromosome. To draw an analogy, our chromosomes are like a library that holds our genetic information and each chromosome pair is one of the individual bookshelves. Each book represents a single gene, and the text of the book is the detailed genetic information cells need to function. Every cell in the body is a library containing over 35,000 books – the current estimate of the number of individual genes human beings possess.

CELL CO-OPERATION

It's clear, therefore, that there is an enormous amount of information stored in the tiny volume of space in each cell. Common sense dictates that for large numbers of cells to co-exist in harmony they would have to obey certain rules. These would include a respect for their neighbours in taking only their fair share of available nutrients such as oxygen and energy-giving glucose from the bloodstream. They would need to respect their own space so that they don't over-reproduce and crowd out the cells next door. Normal cells die and are replaced by new ones during the lifespan of the host, so that's another process that needs to be precisely controlled. All of these rules, and many more, are indeed followed by normal cells and form part of the genetic code. Despite rapid advances in our knowledge of cell control we're still at an early stage of under-standing the whole process.

Generally speaking cancer arises when an abnormality, or mutation, arises in the DNA of at least one cell, which sets it off on a path that no longer acknowledges the rule book of cell behaviour. Usually cancerous cells have an advantage over their neighbours in terms of reproduction speed, in their ability to gain extra nutrition and in the property of invasion, which allows them to take over space that should have been occupied by normal cells. Initially this happens in the immediate surroundings of the abnormal cell but as time goes on the cancer cells spread to more distant parts of the body, transported by the lymphatic system or the bloodstream.

This loss of cell control, resulting in unregulated cancer cell division plus the ability to invade local tissues or spread to distant sites are the hallmarks of cancer.

Jargon terms

Although medical jargon terms can often be substituted by plain English with no loss of meaning it is inevitable that some terms arise quite frequently and are worth knowing about. Doctors sometimes forget that terms they are used to using are quite foreign to non-medics. A few of these are mentioned here and others will be explained as they occur in the book.

TUMOUR

A tumour is a swelling or lump, and that's all the word properly means. The problem is that in layman's language the word tumour is often taken to imply a cancerous lump. Unless a doctor is mindful of this fact he or she can inadvertently cause alarm by referring to a 'tumour' in front of the patient, meaning only that there is a lump. What the patient will take away from the conversation is however that they've got cancer. This may not necessarily be so.

BENIGN

A benign lump (or tumour!) is bigger than the surrounding tissues but it still behaves according to the normal rules of cell behaviour. It is not cancer, nor is it an early stage of cancer. Unless a benign lump is so big it causes problems by its size as such, benign lumps are harmless. There are many causes of benign lumps in the breast, and these are covered in chapter 4.

MALIGNANT

This is an alternative word for cancer. A malignant lump or tumour is one that disobeys all the rules concerning cell behaviour, as described above. Breast cancer is a malignant disease.

METASTASIS

This means spread to a distant site in the body, which is a feature of more advanced cancers. Therefore a breast cancer that has spread to the lymph nodes in the armpit may be said in medical parlance to have 'metastasised' to the lymph nodes. Cancer cells may also be spread by the bloodstream to other more distant regions of the body. Breast cancer shows a tendency to spread, or metastasise, in this way to the bones, lungs, liver and the brain. Metastatic cancer means that cancer has spread in this way, and it is the most serious or advanced type of cancer of the breast or of any other type.

PROGNOSIS

This is an alternative medical word for outlook. A person's prognosis, in respect of cancer, generally means the length of time that they can expect to survive following the diagnosis and after receiving full treatment. More detail on this subject is covered in chapters 5 to 8.

Chapter 2

What Causes Breast Cancer?

This is of course the $64,000 question, and not just for breast cancer. There are no definite answers, but plenty of clues. In general, cancer is caused by abnormalities in our DNA or genetic makeup interacting with the world inside us or the world we live in; the environment. If we accept this theory, which seems accurate, that it is primarily a fault in DNA that leads to the cancer process, then one of the possible causes of breast cancer will be DNA damage from some outside influence.

Radiation

Exposure to excessive radiation is a well-known cause of DNA damage and a recognised cause of all sorts of cancers, notably those of the blood and lymph system, and this has often been observed in practice. For example, the risk of breast cancer was doubled among teenage girls exposed to radiation during the Second World War. Another study of women who had repeated X-rays for tuberculosis (TB) found that there was a risk among women who were first X-rayed between the ages of 10 and 14 years. Fortunately, as mass X-rays for TB are a thing of the past this risk is not relevant today.

Other studies have shown that women with Hodgkin's disease (a form of cancer of the lymph nodes) who received X-ray therapy to the chest as part of the treatment of that condition have an increased risk of breast cancer. The increase in risk depended on the dose of the radiation they received and the age at which they received it.

However, a history of excess radiation exposure, given as radiotherapy, applies to only a tiny minority of the number of women in the UK who develop breast cancer. Ordinary exposure from X-rays (for example a chest X-ray or a mammogram) is not enough to cause significant DNA damage and is therefore not a common cause of breast cancer.

The menstrual cycle effect

One of the most important observations is that breast cancer is more common in women who experience the onset of their periods at an early age (below 15), or who continue having periods until an older age (over 55). During the monthly menstrual cycle there are many hormone changes going on routinely in every woman, most of which also have some effect on breast tissues. With each period the hormone levels are reset and the process goes round again. This repeated stimulation of the breasts may encourage or amplify a fault in the cell growth and repair processes and the more menstrual cycles that a woman has in her life, the more this is likely to occur.

Conversely, women who start their periods late or who have their ovaries removed before the age of 35 have a smaller risk of getting breast cancer. Having your first child early is also protective against breast cancer, leading to the idea that perhaps it is the number of menstrual cycles a woman has before her first pregnancy that is the determining risk factor: the fewer the better.

Specific gene types

In a small number of women specific inherited gene patterns are known to increase the risk of developing breast cancer. These women usually also have a family history of breast cancer and possibly a family history of cancer of the ovary, which appears to share some of the same genetic risk. The two best known of these genes are: BRCA1 and BRCA2. Women who develop breast cancer at a young age (under 40) have a 1 in 4 chance of having the BRCA1 or BRCA2 gene, and the close female relatives of such a woman may benefit from genetic tests and counselling (this issue is covered again in chapter 10). Having the BRCA1 or BRCA2 gene does not mean that you would definitely get breast or any other type of cancer, only that your risk of doing so is above average. To help put it in perspective, only 4 per cent of all breast cancers are actually associated with either of these two gene abnormalities.

Risk factors

In the main we have to set to one side the question of what actually causes breast cancer, because we don't have the knowledge to answer it in other than very broad terms. Nor is it just one cause we're looking for, but many. As with all cancers what seems to matter is the interplay between a person's genetic makeup, which sets to a large extent their inbuilt tendency to getting cancer (or almost any other disease) and their environmental exposure to potential triggers for the disease. Thus someone who has a high genetic risk of developing cancer might still remain disease-free all her life if she never comes across important trigger factors. Equally important but no better understood are the protective factors that can increase our resistance to developing cancer. Knowledge of this would give us the opportunity to be more proactive about our cancer risks. Some information is known on this subject and is also covered in chapter 10.

We can, however, focus more accurately on 'risk factors' for breast cancer. These are associated observations or facts that do not in themselves explain why the cancer occurs, but when present make it more likely that it will arise.

GENDER

Breast cancer is much more common in women than in men, probably related to the monthly changes in hormonal factors such as oestrogen in women. Further information on breast cancer in men is given in chapter 9.

AGE

This is easily the most important risk factor. In terms of numbers of women affected, breast cancer is primarily a disease of older women. At age 30 about 20 women per 100,000 in the UK develop breast cancer. By age 40 about 80 per 100,000 do so and by the average age of the menopause (51) the figure is about 150 per 100,000. Following the menopause the rate of increase slows but still reaches approximately 220 per 100,000 in 80 year-olds.

Putting it another way, approximately a quarter of breast cancers affect women under the age of 50, a half occur in the 20 years between the ages of 50 and 69 and the remaining quarter develop in women who are 70 years or older.

The impact of breast cancer as a cause of death across the age groups presents a different picture, for the simple reason that it is uncommon for younger women to die from any cause, compared to older women. So if you take all women who die at the age of 80 and look at how many of them have died of breast cancer you will see that it is around 2 per cent. Of women who die at the age of 40 the figure is nearly 20 per cent. Breast cancer is thus a relatively common cause of death in women under the age of 50, an age at which they often have strong family commitments.

GEOGRAPHICAL LOCATION

We mentioned earlier that there is about a five-fold difference between the Far East and Western countries in the likelihood of women developing breast cancer. As with some other health measures, Japanese women have a low risk, as do those from the Indian subcontinent. White women in the UK are among those with the highest risk in the world, along with the USA, Canada, New Zealand and most of Scandinavia. In a trend similar to that observed in heart disease, people who move from a country with a low incidence of breast cancer to one with a high incidence tend over just a couple of generations to show this increased risk themselves. This emphasises the importance of factors in the environment, including dietary habits, pollution, levels of exercise and the like. When people adopt the lifestyle of the West, they unfortunately get more than they bargain for.

NUMBER OF MENSTRUAL PERIODS

This was covered above, along with the related risk factor of age at first birth. Women who give birth for the first time after the age of 35 are more than twice as likely to develop breast cancer as those who give birth before they are 20. These older mothers actually have an even higher risk than women who have no children. Women who have a natural menopause after the age of 55 are twice as likely to develop breast cancer as women who experience the menopause before the age of 45.

FAMILY HISTORY

Taking all the genetic factors together, including the presence of the BRCA1 or BRCA2 genes, up to 10 per cent of breast cancer in Western populations may be accounted for by inheritance from one or both parents. Only one of the 23 pairs of chromosomes in human beings determines the sex of a child, and the other 22 pairs are transmitted equally from the mother and the father. The tendency to breast cancer passes through genes in the main group, thus a breast cancer tendency can be passed to a girl from her father as easily as it can from her mother. The same is true of male breast cancer although this is a much less common disease than female breast cancer.

When breast cancer develops secondary to a genetic reason it will usually develop in a younger woman, under 65. Having a first degree relative (mother, sister or daughter) who developed breast cancer before the age of 50 at least doubles a woman's chance of developing breast cancer, and the younger the relative was at the time of diagnosis then the greater the risk. Having two first-degree relatives with breast cancer multiplies the risk even further.

Guidelines to help decide when a woman is at significantly higher than average risk of developing breast cancer on account of her family history are summarised in table 1.

Table 1: Factors increasing the risk of hereditary cancer of the breast

Any one of these categories:

- A first-degree relative with cancer of both breasts or breast and ovarian cancer.
- A first-degree relative diagnosed under 40 or a first-degree male relative with breast cancer diagnosed at any age.
- Two close (first- or second-degree) relatives diagnosed under 60 from the same side of the family.
- Three or more close relatives with breast or ovarian cancer on the same side of the family.

(First-degree female relative = mother, sister, daughter)
(Second-degree = grandmother, granddaughter, aunt, niece)

If you do have a raised risk on these criteria it is important to keep it in context. Remember that most women with a first-degree relative who has breast cancer will not themselves develop the disease (their risk is increased by 5.5 per cent above normal). Conversely, most women with breast cancer have no family history of it.

DIETARY FAT

Although there is a close link between the incidence of breast cancer in a country and the dietary fat intake in that country, more detailed studies have not shown a particularly strong or consistent relationship between fat intake in any individual and their risk of developing breast cancer. It's possible that instead of a high fat intake being a risk factor for breast cancer instead it is a protective factor in certain diets, absent in high fat diets, which reduces the risk of breast cancer in those who eat it. A possibility for this protective factor is the natural plant oestrogens (called phyto-estrogens) present in high concentration in plant sources such as soy. This could possibly explain the reduced rate of breast cancer seen in Japanese and similar populations where the phytoestrogen content of their diet can be several hundred times higher than in Western diets.

WEIGHT

Being overweight is associated with a doubling of the risk of breast cancer in women who are past the menopause. However, among pre-menopausal women obesity is associated with reduced breast cancer incidence. The link is not well understood but fatty tissue is known to convert some of the body's natural steroids into oestrogen. Post-menopausal women, by definition, produce less oestrogen from their ovaries. If instead they produce oestrogen from fatty tissue this means that they extend the time during which they have a higher level of oestrogen circulating in the blood. As we'll come to later, certain types of breast cancer are sensitive to oestrogen so may be more prone to develop if there is more of this hormone around over a longer part of a woman's life.

ALCOHOL INTAKE

Some studies have shown a link between the amount of alcohol people drink and the incidence of breast cancer, but this relationship is not consistent and may be influenced by other factors rather than alcohol. For example, people with a very high alcohol intake tend to eat a poor diet, low in fruit and vegetables. Fruit and vegetables contain anti-oxidants, which are compounds that can mop up other highly active chemicals called free radicals. Free radicals are normal by-products of the body's use of oxygen as a fuel, but they are capable of damaging some of the more sensitive chemical processes that go on in cells. We therefore have inbuilt natural ways of dealing with free radicals but if these are overwhelmed then we rely on our dietary intake of extra anti-oxidants to cope.

A normal healthy diet contains plenty of anti-oxidants, and is protective against many cancers, including that of the breast. The poor diet of an alcoholic may be the real link with breast cancer rather than a direct toxic effect of alcohol on the breast.

SMOKING

Smoking used to be thought not to influence the likelihood of developing breast cancer, but recent research shows this is not the case. Smoking does increase the risk of breast cancer but because it tends to make the menopause occur sooner this has a balancing effect that has tended to mask the increased risk.

HORMONE TREATMENTS

This is an important issue and deserves a section to itself. Women commonly take hormones in two forms: as the oral contraceptive pill and as hormone replacement therapy (HRT) to alleviate the symptoms of the menopause. The hormones within these preparations are designed to mimic the effects of the natural 'female hormones', oestrogen and progesterone, although the amounts of hormones used in contraception are about three or four times more potent than those in HRT.

Oral contraceptives

There are two types of oral contraceptive. The standard 'combined' pill contains both oestrogen and progesterone-like components, whereas the 'mini-pill' contains only the progesterone-like hormone. Both types are associated with a small increase in the risk of developing breast cancer (1.24 times greater than women who have not used oral contraceptives). This excess risk fades to zero by 10 years after stopping the oral contraceptives.

On the positive side, cancers diagnosed in women taking the oral contraceptive pill are less likely to have spread than those cancers diagnosed in women who have never used the oral contraceptive. It also appears that oral contraceptives reduce the risk of a woman later developing cancer of the lining of the womb or of the ovary. These positive factors cancel out the slight excess of breast cancer risk, so that in examining populations as a whole one sees no increase in mortality from breast cancer in contraceptive users.

Hormone replacement therapy

HRT taken for many years has been known for some time to increase the risk of breast cancer. The risk increases with the length of time that HRT is used and becomes detectable after about five years of treatment. The risk falls once HRT is stopped, and takes about five years to drop back to the average in the population.

Stating the breast cancer risk another way to illustrate this, in women aged 50 who do not use HRT about 45 in every thousand will be diagnosed with breast cancer by the time they reach the age of 70. In women who start HRT at age 50 and use it for five years the figure would be 47 women developing breast cancer in every thousand. In those who take HRT for 10 years, breast cancer will occur in 51 in a thousand and for 15 years it will be 57 in a thousand.

The best presently available evidence tells us that breast cancers that occur in women taking HRT are smaller, less advanced and of a more treatable type than breast cancers occurring in women not taking HRT. This accounts for the fact that despite the increased numbers of cancers arising due to HRT, the actual mortality of women from breast cancer is the same in the HRT and non-HRT populations. Some breast cancer experts feel, however, that the balance of risk has swung against HRT given for longer than five years. As is made clear next, there are additional factors to consider with HRT.

Other breast problems related to HRT

Women in the pre-menopause who take HRT often get breast pain and benign breast lumps, including cysts (fluid-filled lumps). HRT may cause benign breast lumps that are already present to get bigger. In the UK we place great emphasis not only on the need for a woman to check her breasts regularly and report any changes to her doctor but also we have a national screening service that offers periodic mammograms to women over 50. HRT is known to increase the density of breast tissue, which makes it harder for the X-rays used in mammography to penetrate the breast. It is therefore of concern that HRT can make it more difficult to detect breast cancer by mammography.

HRT is very much a hot topic at the moment, particularly because the results of recent large research studies have shown that it is not as beneficial as previously thought in protecting women against developing hardening of the arteries, heart disease and strokes. HRT can, however, have beneficial effects on preventing bone thinning (osteoporosis) and reducing symptoms of the menopause such as hot flushes. More detail on the pros and cons of HRT is in the companion book in this series, on the menopause.

PREVIOUS BENIGN BREAST DISEASE

Some types of pre-existing breast disease, although benign in themselves, are associated with an increased risk of developing breast cancer. The exact description of the type of breast disease this refers to is quite technical but it is due to heaping up of the cells that line the ductules leading from the milk-producing lobules. The name for this condition is severe atypical epithelial hyperplasia. (As with most medical jargon terms this isn't quite so complex once it's broken down into its components. 'Atypical' means different from the normal. 'Epithelial' just means that it concerns the lining cells, as the word 'epithelium' is the technical one for 'skin' or 'lining'. 'Hyperplasia' means overgrowth.) When severe atypical hyperplasia is present it increases a woman's chance of later developing breast cancer by about four times. If she also has a first-degree relative with breast cancer then her risk doubles again to about nine fold, so it is a significant finding.

The symptom of this condition is that of a breast lump and, as we cover in the next two chapters, there are many potential causes of lumps. Finding out exactly what is the cause of a lump is of course part of the proper process of managing breast conditions in general. For this to happen it's essential for a woman to be aware of her breasts and report changes early. Fortunately most women now have the confidence to come forward early on finding a lump and have it properly checked out.

There are some other types of benign breast lump that are associated with small increases in breast cancer risk. These are also covered in the next chapter.

Influencing breast cancer risk

It will be clear from what's been said so far that we don't know a lot about what actually causes breast cancer to occur. It will also be clear that a lot of the risk factors are not readily modifiable. We certainly can't stop ourselves getting older, re-choose our parents or pick the ages at which menstruation starts and stops. And there must be very few women indeed who plan their first pregnancy specifically on the basis of risk reduction for breast cancer in later life. To a certain extent it might therefore seem that a woman's destiny as far as breast cancer is concerned is mapped out for her at an early age and that there's not much she can do about her risk. For several reasons this is incorrect.

First, some of the risk factors *are* modifiable. Obesity, smoking and excess alcohol intake are entirely under personal control. Moreover, improvements in these three factors have knock-on benefits to health in other respects. Obesity is associated with a raised risk of other cancers such as of the colon and bowel and increases the chance of getting high blood pressure, heart disease and diabetes. Smoking causes lung cancer, heart disease and narrowing of arteries elsewhere in the body. A modest alcohol intake (about one unit daily, equivalent to a standard glass of wine) lowers the risk of getting heart disease but higher consumption than this is more likely to lead to ill health. Despite the difficulty in proving it unconditionally, all health experts are agreed that an increased intake of fruit and vegetables in our diet lowers our general risk of getting cancer as well as reducing the risk of heart disease – the big killers of those who live in the West.

In other words a healthy lifestyle, combined with adequate and regular exercise, makes a positive contribution to lowering the risk of breast cancer as well as improving general health.

Second is the impact of breast cancer screening. The mortality associated with breast cancer in women who undergo mammography screening is approximately 40 per cent less than those who do not. Breast cancer screening is dealt with in more detail shortly, but the message here is that participation is very helpful. We have to do more to ensure that a greater percentage of the population make use of this facility.

Third is the increasing evidence that breast cancer risk can be reduced by hormone treatment that blocks the action of oestrogen in certain ways. This important subject is expanded upon in chapters 6 to 8. It is an expanding field of medical research and is very likely to produce more in the way of drugs that can protect against breast cancer within the next few years.

Fourth is the fact that we are not standing still in the search for natural ways to enhance our resistance to breast cancer. For example, trials are underway to look at the effect of selenium, a trace element present naturally in our diet and which is thought to have cancer-preventing properties. Selenium is a component of several anti-oxidant compounds, which may account for any such power. It is present in high concentration in seaweed, which is a significant element of the Japanese diet and so offers an alternative explanation why Japanese women have a low breast cancer risk.

It will be some years yet before we have reliable answers to which of the diet and lifestyle changes we can make have the most effect. Compared to analysing the effect of a drug, which can be carefully manufactured and controlled in dosage, diet and lifestyle studies are much more difficult to do. There are so many possible variables to consider, large numbers of people behaving in a consistent way over years are needed to observe differences between groups, and the studies are expensive to conduct. Such funding has to come from public sources, as without a drug to test the pharmaceutical companies have no interest. One of the questions such studies need to answer is not only whether dietary supplements are effective, but also what is the optimum dose to take. There are concerns that over-use of vitamins and supplements can lead to as many or more problems than they might solve.

Chapter 3

Examining the Breasts

Before we get into the finer detail of what types of breast cancer there are, and indeed what are the alternative causes of breast lumps and other breast-related symptoms we should clarify what a woman needs to know in order to check her breasts, and what to expect at a breast clinic.

There are three areas of relevant information here:

1 self-examination of the breasts
2 screening for breast cancer
3 tests used by specialists

1. Self-examination of the breasts

Although it seems to make common sense that regular self-examination of the breasts should be a good thing to do it is still a controversial subject, with pros and cons. A lump in the breast is the first sign of the disease in up to 90 per cent of women who have breast cancer, but lumps in the breasts are very common, and 80 per cent of them are not cancerous. You could say that a disadvantage of regularly looking for lumps is that you will find them, and although the statistics are in favour of such lumps being harmless much worry, and sometimes unnecessary tests such as tissue samples (biopsies – see shortly) may be done in the process of proving them to be so.

In reality many women find it difficult to be sure what's a lump and what's not. That should never hold them back from going along to their doctor to have it checked out, but in practice it does.

Being 'breast aware' implies that what you are trying to do is to become familiar with what's normal for you, and to report any changes as soon as you find them. For example, some women notice that they have lumps that disappear and reappear during the course of their monthly cycles and others do not. Both situations are equally normal. Once you know what your own pattern is then you can become more adept at noticing a change.

WHAT TO LOOK FOR
It's much easier to feel the breasts while in the bath or the shower and with a soapy hand and also to have a routine of inspecting them in the mirror.

The sort of things to look out for are:

- any new lump or thickening of the breast tissue
- anything new about their appearance

Figure 3: Breast self-examination

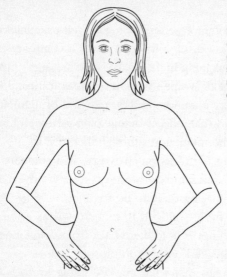

Stand before a mirror, hands on hips. Look for any lumps, difference in size or shape, skin dimpling, change in nipple shape or nipple discharge.

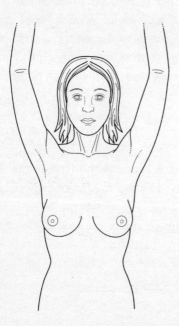

Re-inspect with arms held high. Make sure you check below and the sides of your breasts.

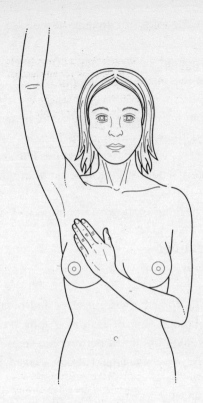

Use plenty of soap and water in the shower to lubricate your hands and feel all areas of the breasts as before. Remember to check up towards the armpits too.

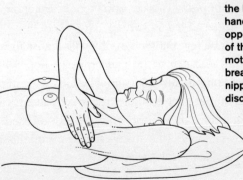

Lie flat, with one hand behind your head to spread the breast. With the other hand, feel all over the opposite breast. Use the flat of the hand and a circular motion. Repeat for the other breast. Gently squeeze the nipples to check for any discharge.

- any skin changes (particularly dimples or crinkling of the skin or discolouration)
- pain that you're not used to getting
- discharge from or changes in the shape of the nipple

To get the most information from inspecting your breasts remember that by raising your arms, and thereby moving the muscles and connecting tissues under the breasts, you can reveal features like skin dimpling that you might not see if you just look face on with your arms by your side every time.

A suggested routine of self-checking is shown in figure 3.

2. Screening for breast cancer

MAMMOGRAPHY

The dominant method of looking for otherwise unsuspected breast cancer is by low-dose X-ray photography, or mammography. Previously this was offered to all women in the UK between the ages of 50 and 64 every three years but the upper age limit of routine screening is currently being extended to 70 years.

The technique is quite simple, but can be uncomfortable. Each breast has to be briefly squeezed to flatten it between two clear plastic sheets, whereupon the X-ray is taken and then the other breast is done.

When a breast lump can be felt, mammography will almost always be able to confirm the appearance to be cancerous or not. When mammography detects an abnormality that cannot be felt on examination then it is only about 50 per cent accurate in correctly identifying breast cancer. Mammography is never the only procedure used to make a diagnosis of breast cancer. This always has to include tissue sampling of some type (see later in this chapter).

Roles of mammography

Mammography is useful not just as a population screening tool for the detection of breast cancer. It's also helpful in:

- *The accurate location of a cancer*
  By taking two films from different angles a precise location of an abnormality can be pinpointed. When necessary this can allow the specialist to place a thin wire locator exactly at the right spot, which is followed down to the cancer when it is being removed at operation.
- *Checking for other cancers*
  It is possible for more than one cancer to exist at the same time, in either the same or the other breast. Modern surgical techniques aim to preserve as much of the normal breast as possible, but in doing so one has to be certain that a small overlooked cancer elsewhere is not being left behind.
- *Follow up*
  In women who have had breast cancer treatment mammography may be used to watch out for the reappearance of cancer at the original site or elsewhere in the same or the other breast.

Effectiveness of mammography

Mammography too has had its critics, but there is equally eminent medical opinion that states it is both worthwhile and effective at reducing the mortality from breast cancer. Critics suggest that although it sounds impressive to say that the early detection of breast cancer through screening may reduce breast cancer deaths by somewhere between 25 and 50 per cent, what this means in reality is that one woman's life will be saved for every 1000 women screened over a period of 10 years. Expert or not, we can all have our own opinion on whether that much effort represents a good use of resources and medical manpower. Most women will have no difficulty in reaching a decision.

Another side of the debate concerns the age range of women selected for screening and the frequency of screening. In the USA routine screening is now recommended for women over 40. Younger women have denser breast tissue, which requires slightly more exposure from X-rays to produce the mammogram as well as making it harder to detect cancer changes. As their breasts change more rapidly an increased frequency of screening is required, down to perhaps yearly or every 18 months.

Changing the breast screening service in the UK in such a way would have very large implications for the cost of the service, for the amount of resources it would take and the availability of manpower to accurately do high quality screening. This is another of the objections made by mammography critics, who would like more money put into breast cancer research. The problem is of course that both points of view are valid. We already know that the three-year spacing between mammograms that is the current UK practice is enough of a gap for some women to develop breast cancer in the intervening time, and sometimes these are fast growing cancers that have spread by the time the next mammogram is done. We also know that many women who do not currently attend for screening are from the less well-off sections of society, or are from ethnic minority groups, many of whom have poor medical access or uptake in other health areas too.

Most of all, the many funding shortfalls of the NHS are dealt with by financial decisions that are taken largely outside the public arena and as the issues are of a highly technical nature we have to rely heavily on medical authority providing clear guidance and politicians providing enough funds to make it all happen. Neither is reliably the case.

In the meantime we need to accept that mammography, although imperfect, is the best tool we have for breast cancer screening. If we increase the percentage of women who make use of it and combine it with better self-awareness and willingness to report changes as soon as they appear then, in combination with the fact that we do have excellent breast cancer specialists and treatment facilities in the UK, the outlook for women in respect of breast cancer will continue to improve.

3. Tests used by specialists

ULTRASOUND

Ultrasound is high frequency sound waves and a familiar technique to most women who have had a baby in the past 25 years or so. The same type of instrument that can give clear pictures of the baby in the womb is also widely used to gain information about the other structures under the skin, including breast tissue. Ultrasound is particularly good at detecting the presence of fluid, which is the constituent of breast cysts. The vast majority of breast cysts are benign and can be confirmed so by removing fluid from the cyst by a needle and syringe. The fluid thus obtained is then sent for microscopic analysis to check that the cells floating in the fluid are not cancerous (see 'cytology' below). An experienced clinician will often be able to decide that a lump is due to a cyst just by examining it, but ultrasound will confirm a cyst before the attempt at withdrawing fluid.

Ultrasound is painless and completely harmless – it uses no radiation. Presently its main use is as a tool to help assess palpable breast lumps. Its usefulness as a screening tool is still uncertain although it is being researched, particularly in younger women in whom the breast tissue is denser and who are more prone to have lumpy breasts in any case.

MAGNETIC RESONANCE SCANS

Magnetic resonance scanning (MRI) is one of the relatively new ways in which detailed images of the inside of the body can be obtained without causing any harm to the patient. To conduct an MRI scan the patient is placed within the magnetic field produced by a large circular magnet. The field is rapidly switched on and off, which causes the water molecules within the body to emit radio waves. Detectors within the scanner pick up these signals from the tissues and computers convert this information into images. Breast MRI scanning is not currently a routine service in the UK. However, MRI can give very clear images and contribute to the information available to the breast cancer specialist prior to planning treatment.

EXAMINATION OF BREAST CELLS

Whereas ultrasound and MRI scanning have a variable degree of availability across different regions of the country and are perhaps of debatable benefit, certain other tests are always part of the range of tests in common use in breast cancer specialist centres. Examination of cells from the breast is one of these. Cells from breast cancer look, to the experienced eye, different to those from ordinary breast tissue or benign breast lumps. The advantage of cell examination is that it can confirm a diagnosis of either a benign or a cancerous breast lump using techniques that need very little in the way of tissue material for inspection. An experienced breast specialist can obtain a sufficient number of cells using just a syringe and needle inserted into a lump, which also involves very little trauma to the woman having the test and takes seconds to perform. Alternatively, if the problem is a nipple discharge, then examining some of the nipple fluid placed on a glass slide can be very useful to see if there is an underlying cancer.

The technique of examining cells from a fine needle test or nipple discharge is called cytology. Although it is possible to use the sorts of needles and syringes that a doctor would normally use for taking blood samples there are also very thin needles used that are more suitable for reaching lumps deep within the breast tissue. Often this is referred to as fine needle aspiration cytology, or FNAC for short.

There are three ways in which breast cells or tissues can be obtained for examination:

1 By examining cells drawn from a solid breast lump or a cyst using a syringe and needle as described above. The tiny amount removed by the needle from a lump can be spread on glass slides and examined within minutes to check for any abnormality. The fluid obtained from benign breast cysts is usually slightly murky, but not bloodstained. Bloodstained fluid can also be the direct result of trauma from the needle if it's been necessary to probe around a little bit with the needle to get the tip in the right place, so it doesn't necessarily mean there's a problem. Bloodstained fluid is therefore always sent for analysis. If breast cyst fluid contains no obvious blood and the lump disappears when it has been drained it is usually safe to say that the cyst is benign. In those circumstances a breast cancer specialist may recommend that no further treatment is required. Some GPs do have experience of draining breast cysts (it is a fairly easy technique to learn and does not need specialised equipment) but it would still be necessary for a woman with a breast cyst to see a breast cancer specialist unless the specialist knew her already and had agreed with the GP that drainage was a sufficient course of action.

2 By removing a more substantial specimen of breast tissue using a needle specially designed to remove a core of breast tissue. This is done under local anaesthetic and the total amount of tissue removed is very small; about the size of the tip of a Biro pen. Several such samples, known as core biopsies, can be taken from a single area of suspicious breast tissue to increase the chance of detecting an

abnormality. These are then fixed in preservative and cast in wax blocks before sections of the tissue are looked at under the microscope.

3 By removing the lump en masse. This is called open biopsy, and involves a local or general anaesthetic. Open biopsy is only undertaken once the simpler investigations such as cytology and/or core biopsy have been performed; one would not usually do it as a first step in diagnosing the exact nature of a breast lump. Even then it is only used if these primary investigations have left some doubt as to the exact nature of the lump. Open biopsy allows the lump to be completely removed, which therefore allows complete analysis, and at the same time it removes the abnormal tissue, which can then be examined just like the tissue removed by core biopsy. Should it therefore prove to be a cancer then the process of removing it has already been done.

Triple assessment

This refers to the combination of clinical examination of the breasts by an expert, plus the results of investigations such as mammography, plus the results of breast cell or tissue examination. In the hands of a specialist the combination of all three means that a confident diagnosis of breast cancer or benign breast disease can be made in close to 100 per cent of women.

Concerning clinical examination, the most important pointers that a specialist looks for in examining a woman newly referred to the breast clinic are:

- signs that breast cancer is present
- signs that the cancer has spread

SIGNS OF BREAST CANCER

Ultimately cancer has to be proven by examining abnormal tissue under the microscope but in the course of initially examining a woman with a breast lump the specialist looks for certain clues that might indicate a malignant rather than a benign cause. First the shape and symmetry of the breasts is inspected with the woman sitting, arms by her side and then with the arms upraised, to stretch the underlying muscles. Pressing her hands on her hips is an additional way of tensing the chest wall muscles in order to reveal any changes in shape that can be less obvious when the muscles are relaxed. To feel the breast tissue the woman is usually asked to lie on her back with her hands tucked behind her head, again to tighten the underlying muscles, and then the doctor feels the breast tissue in a methodical way with the flat of the hand or the fingertips. Certain findings point towards a diagnosis of cancer if they are present, but they can also occur in benign breast disease, thus:

Dimpling of the skin

Breast cancer tends to tether the overlying skin and draw it inwards. This might not be immediately obvious, but can become so when the arms are in different positions. Skin dimpling can also occur over benign breast problems such as breast infection.

Inversion of the nipple

This is not the same as a retracted nipple, which is a fairly common problem and gives a slit-like appearance that can cause problems in breastfeeding but is otherwise harmless. Inversion of the nipple is where the whole nipple is drawn inwards. Cancer of the breast is not the only cause; it also occurs in benign breast disease.

Orange-peel skin

In this condition, which is often referred to in medical parlance by the French phrase *peau d'orange*, the skin of the breast has a pitted surface very much like the skin of an orange. It is due to blockage of the lymph drainage within the breast and is usually associated with advanced breast cancer.

Bloodstained nipple discharge

Ninety per cent of bloodstained nipple discharge will be found to be due to benign breast problems. As you will remember from earlier in the book approximately 20 milk ducts open on the surface of the nipple and if there is discharge from more than one then it is highly likely that it is due to the normal discharge of fluid that occurs in many women even when they are not breastfeeding. Breast cancer tends to occur in only one segment of the breast, so a bloodstained discharge coming from only a single duct on the nipple, indicating that it arises from only one segment of the breast, would be regarded with more suspicion.

There are other findings that might be present on examining the breasts of a woman with a lump. There might be a visible swelling or a difference in size in the breasts or they might simply not look the same in comparison with each other. These features would, however, simply be the result of having a breast lump and would not indicate one way or another if the lump were benign or malignant.

Signs of cancer spread

The specialist is mainly interested in finding out if the cancer has spread to the lymph nodes. (The lymph drainage of the breasts was described in chapter 1, and is illustrated in figure 2.) The doctor can examine the axillary (armpit) nodes by supporting the woman's arm (to let the arm muscles relax) and then sweeping his or her fingers around the space between the upper arm and the ribs. Nodes may also be felt along the line between the breast and the armpit, where the 'tail' of the breast extends. The other important area examined is in the hollow behind the collar bone, specifically at the angle between the collar bone and the muscles of the neck (see figure 2).

When a lymph node contains cancer cells it may swell enough to become palpable. Generally speaking lymph from the breast drains first to the nodes under the armpit, then to the group closer to the collar bone, and then on to the nodes above the collar bone and beside the neck muscles. It's a generalisation but the presence of cancer-containing nodes in these second and third positions indicates that the cancer is at a more advanced stage than if the only involved lymph nodes are those in the armpit.

We'll later cover in more detail the procedure of locating and removing lymph nodes, which is sometimes done as part of the assessment and treatment of breast cancer. Microscopic inspection of nodes obtained this way allows the pathologist to detect small numbers of cancer cells that haven't yet caused the node to obviously enlarge or be palpable.

Tests for distant spread of cancer

The concept of breast cancer initially being confined to a single primary site in the breast, growing over a period of time and at some later date spreading in an organised way first to the axillary lymph nodes, and later to other nodes is neater than occurs in reality. Breast cancer can spread via the bloodstream rather than the lymph system and reach virtually any other part of the body.

Similarly the lymph nodes are not perfect traps capable of catching every migrating cancer cell without fail. Sometimes it's found that the neck lymph nodes contain cancer cells with little or no evidence of involved nodes in the armpit. There are also other, much less usual, routes of lymph drainage of the breast to regions within the chest or abdomen, which are much harder to detect with clinical examination.

The potential of breast cancer to spread is not equal in all women. Most cancers that have the potential to spread do so relatively early on in the course of the disease, and so it can happen even with what seems like a small breast cancer that's been investigated as soon as a woman has become aware of it, that it has already spread. Common sites of distant spread of breast cancer are the bones (anywhere, but especially the spine), the liver, lungs and the brain.

One of the important steps in completing the initial assessment of a woman who has breast cancer is therefore to detect if there has already been distant spread. Sometimes there will be clues this has happened from a woman's symptoms, such as for example the presence of recent onset back pain which on X-ray then appears to be from a deposit of cancer cells within the spine. Or the blood tests that are part of every woman's investigation may show abnormal levels of enzymes (chemicals) that come from the liver, indicating the possibility of a spread (metastasis) there. Scans such as ultrasound, magnetic resonance imaging (MRI), CT (computerised X-rays that give a cross-section picture of the body) or bone scans (which use a small amount of radioactive material that's picked up by bone metastases and shows up on a special camera) can all be used to confirm the presence or absence of spread.

When distant spread has occurred the aims of treatment have to be modified accordingly. Generally speaking distant spread is associated with a shorter outlook thereafter. It's not good news.

Assessing how far a cancer has already developed at the time it's diagnosed is called staging, and we'll return to the effect staging has upon the available treatment choices.

Receptor status

One of the most important differences in the nature of breast cancer cells between different women is whether the cells are sensitive to hormone influence. To put this into more understandable terms a brief diversion into what hormones are, and how they work, is useful.

HORMONES

A hormone is a substance produced in one part of the body that has its effect in another part of the body, which it reaches via the bloodstream. There are many important hormones, such as insulin produced by the pancreas gland inside the abdomen, which controls the level of glucose (sugar) in the blood. The thyroid gland in the neck produces a hormone that regulates the pace of metabolism throughout the body. Steroid hormones produced by the adrenal glands (small pieces of specialised tissue situated above the kidneys) help regulate our blood pressure and salt balance. The list is a long one but our interest in breast cancer mostly concerns the main 'female hormone', oestrogen, which is produced in pre-menopausal women by the ovaries located either side of the womb. In post-menopausal women the oestrogen output from the ovaries falls to nil, but the hormone continues to be made, notably by fatty tissue.

Hormones target certain cells of the body and are able to control them. They do this because of what are called receptor molecules that are present on the surface of the target cells. If we could magnify a hormone molecule sufficiently we'd see that it has a specific shape, and we'd see also that a receptor molecule has a specific complementary shape designed to latch on to the hormone. It's very much like a lock and key situation, in which the hormone is the key, floating around in the bloodstream until it meets the lock that's designed to accept it. When the hormone attaches to the receptor signals are then sent to the cell on which the receptor is placed, thus triggering the cell processes that the hormone is designed to control.

We now know that not all breast cancers are the same in their type and degree of hormone sensitivity, and it's possible to sort cancers into which receptors they are sensitive to, or not as the case may be. This has moved us along a great deal in understanding breast cancer, and how to tackle it. Two types of hormone receptors are of particular importance:

1 Receptors for oestrogen. Breast cancers that are sensitive to oestrogen are called 'oestrogen receptor positive', or 'ER +ve' (adopting the American spelling of estrogen). Receptors for the other main female hormone, progesterone, may also be important but appear secondary to oestrogen receptor status.
2 Receptors for growth factors. Growth factors are, as the name suggests, hormones that stimulate cell and cancer growth. The specific growth factor important in breast cancer is called human epidermal growth factor receptor 2, or HER-2.

It's not known why some breast tumours have these receptors while others do not, but their presence or absence is associated with important differences in their behaviour and in the sort of treatment one can use against them.

OESTROGEN RECEPTORS AND BREAST CANCER

If a breast cancer is ER +ve then this means it can be stimulated by oestrogen. Treatment to remove oestrogen or block its effect should therefore be expected to stop or slow the growth of the tumour. This is exactly what is seen in practice. Drugs that block the effect of oestrogen or that reduce the body's ability to manufacture oestrogen have been shown to delay the growth of breast cancer and improve survival in women with ER +ve disease. More detail on these drugs is in chapters 6 and 7 and in appendix B. Surgical removal of the ovaries (which is nowadays usually done with 'keyhole' techniques) from pre-menopausal women removes most of the source of oestrogen and this too is effective against breast cancer in the same way. It's also possible to shut down the ovaries using drug therapy or X-rays thus avoiding surgery. These anti-oestrogen measures are ineffective if the breast cancer is not sensitive to oestrogen, i.e. is ER −ve.

Concerning other hormones such as growth factors, new treatments are emerging that can block their action. Trastuzumab is an antibody that latches on to HER-2 on the cancer cells and inactivates it. Antibodies are proteins normally produced by our immune system and which are tailored to attack foreign proteins. The development of antibodies as treatments is one of the innovations that the new biotechnologies have made possible.

The presence or absence of hormone receptors on breast cancer cells is helpful to the breast cancer specialist in predicting the likelihood of response to treatments. The details of how this information is used is quite specialised and not covered further here. It's also an area of knowledge that's changing quite quickly. Oestrogen receptors are, however, of established importance, and are the main ones to know about.

Chapter 4

Breast Lumps and Other Symptoms

Breast lumps always cause alarm when they are first found, even though the statistics are strongly in favour of a benign cause. Understandably every woman assumes a lump is cancer until proven otherwise. It's now a national requirement in the UK that a woman with suspected breast cancer will be assessed by a fully trained specialist in breast disease, and the waiting times for such clinics are short. As breast lumps and other breast-related symptoms are common, GPs are also familiar with their preliminary assessment and management. Although a GP may refer a woman to a breast clinic to have the diagnosis of a benign breast lump confirmed he or she will often be able to reassure a woman initially. There are, however, very few situations in which it is appropriate for a GP to deal with a breast lump without specialist referral.

When should a hospital specialist be consulted?

There are now clear guidelines set out for doctors to follow to ensure that all breast problems are dealt with to a uniformly high standard. The following symptoms or findings always merit a referral to a hospital specialist:

- any new breast lump, whether completely new or in an area of pre-existing lumpiness
- lumpiness that's not equal in both breasts and which doesn't disappear after a period
- cysts (see below) that keep recurring
- a breast infection or abscess that doesn't clear up quickly with antibiotics
- pain especially if persistent and in only one breast or if causing a lot of trouble
- nipple discharge in all women over 50
- nipple discharge in women under 50 if there is blood or it appears to come from only one duct on the nipple surface
- distortion of the nipple or of the shape of the breasts
- if a woman appears to have a strong family history of breast cancer (see table 1, page 20) and is looking for advice on her level of risk

The types of breast lumps

Although any type of breast lump can appear at any age, there tend to be different patterns of benign lumps found in younger versus older women. Many young women (under 30) have either generally lumpy (nodular) breasts or have more definite lumps of breast tissue called fibroadenomas. A fibroadenoma is a collection of breast tissue derived from the milk-producing glands (lobules) through which is mixed a variable amount of the tough supporting tissues. In women below 20 years over half of breast lumps are caused by fibroadenomas.

In breastfeeding women a breast abscess is usually easily diagnosed. It causes a lump and local redness and tenderness to appear over a short period of time in one breast. There may be a discharge of pus from the nipple. A minor abscess may resolve spontaneously with continued expression of milk and probably the use of antibiotics but a large abscess may need to be surgically drained with a small cut into the abscess, which lets out the pus.

A cyst is a collection of fluid anywhere in the body. In the breasts cysts can quite easily develop within the duct system, which is after all designed to produce milk. They are commonest in women a few years either side of the menopause. Ultrasound is excellent at confirming a cyst (though they do show up on mammograms too) and often a cyst can be dealt with completely by draining with a syringe and needle. Some women are prone to recurring breast cysts.

There is a miscellaneous number of other benign breast conditions in which lumps or thickening of breast tissue occur. The diagnosis of all breast lumps is along the lines already described: a combination of clinical assessment by a specialist, plus investigations such as mammography and/or ultrasound and tissue sampling.

Breast pain

Breast pain (mastalgia) is one of the commonest symptoms experienced by almost all women at some time. Its severity usually dictates what action a woman will wish to take. If limited to mild discomfort occurring a few days a month in a woman still having regular periods she may opt to do nothing other than accept it as one of life's hassles. Mastalgia can, however, be a miserable and disruptive condition when it persists or is severe. It's uncommon for breast pain to be the sole symptom of breast cancer, but its presence can generate anxiety about breast cancer and this is often the reason why a woman will seek advice about it. Having it confirmed that the condition is benign may be all that's needed in the way of treatment. A few words about breast pain may be useful, as the problem is so common.

Two patterns of breast pain are recognised:

1 Cyclical breast pain. This is the type that comes and goes with the menstrual cycle. It is assumed to be due to hormone fluctuations although there are no obvious differences in hormone levels in women who get cyclical mastalgia compared with those who don't.
2 Non-cyclical mastalgia. This has no pattern, or is always present. It occurs in older women, although they may still be young enough to be having regular periods.

Distinguishing the two types of pain is not so difficult if a woman keeps a diary for a couple of months, in which she records the severity of pain each day. There is some merit in making the distinction as there are slight differences in the approach to treatment in the two types.

CYCLICAL BREAST PAIN TREATMENT

Despite the attractiveness of the concept, hormone treatments show no consistent pattern of results. Some women on the contraceptive pill or on HRT get more breast pain, others get less and there are no brands of either type of medicine that are worse or better than any other. Evening Primrose Oil has been tried over several years without any convincing evidence of benefit, and for this reason has been withdrawn from NHS prescription. It is still available directly from a pharmacy or health store and there are some women who undoubtedly feel it helps them, but not enough to make a good scientific case. It has the distinct advantage of being completely safe and as it is sourced from a 'natural' product many women will still wish to try it first.

Prescription medicines for cyclical mastalgia are available and may be necessary when the symptoms are severe but they have many potential side effects (see bromocriptine and danazol in appendix B).

NON-CYCLICAL BREAST PAIN TREATMENT

This depends to a large extent on what is causing the pain. Whereas cyclical breast pain is probably hormonal, even if we can't prove it, non-cyclical pain could arise from various possible sources. Arthritis of the spine could, for example, nip the nerves that travel from the spinal cord around to the front of the chest. The pain may be felt in the breast area but actually arises from the spine: a situation very similar to leg pains caused by disc trouble in the lower back (sciatica). A small number of women have a well-localised area of pain in one breast that will sometimes respond to a local steroid injection. Most of the time breast pain of benign cause is best treated with a well-fitting bra (which may be worn at night to provide additional support), avoiding caffeine-containing drinks (since caffeine may make breast pain worse) and fatty foods. Some women also gain benefit with ordinary painkillers or anti-inflammatory drugs (like ibuprofen).

BREAST CANCER PAIN

Pain is not usually a big problem with breast cancer and if it does arise it can be controlled. Exactly what sort of treatment is needed depends again on what's causing the pain. If it's coming directly from the cancer area in the breast then oral painkillers will suffice most of the time. However, the strength of those used has to match the level of the pain. Combinations of painkillers with other drugs such as anti-inflammatories can increase the level of pain relief while minimising side effects. In addition there are medicines that affect the way nerves transmit pain (such as amitriptyline and gabapentin). Portable electrical nerve stimulators (TENS machines – transcutaneous electrical nerve stimulators), which apply a small electric current through sticky skin pads can distract the nerves that transmit pain. Alternatively a pulse of radiotherapy to a painful site can also greatly reduce a localised painful site.

A great deal of know-how exists concerning pain management nowadays, especially that caused by cancer. The GP can call upon the expertise of the breast cancer team and the local expert in palliative care for help in this and all other aspects of cancer care as and when required, so there is never any need for a patient to suffer a symptom that potentially can be helped with the right combination of drugs or other forms of treatment.

Chapter 5

The Grades and Stages of Breast Cancer

'Breast cancer' is actually an umbrella term for over 20 different types of cancer that arise from the breast. The majority develop within the milk-producing lobules and/or their associated ductules. These are called 'lobular' or 'ductal' cancers respectively. Only rarely does breast cancer arise from the cells that make up the supporting tissues in between the lobules and ductules.

Grade of cancer

Most of the normal cells of the body replace themselves naturally as time goes by. Some cells, such as skin and the blood cells in the bone marrow, are made quickly but generally the pace of cell renewal is quite slow. Also, when one looks down the microscope at normal cells one sees a highly organised arrangement in which each cell has its place. Cancer cells multiply much faster than normal cells and they tend also to become disorganised. Examining a sample of breast cancer tissue under the microscope allows a pathologist to make an assessment of these features, which can be brought together to make a scoring system of the cancer, called the grade. Three grades are usually described:

1 Grade 1 cells are similar in nature and appearance to normal cells.
2 Grade 2 cells are more abnormal but not grossly so.
3 Grade 3 cells are grossly abnormal. They are aggressive in nature and are more likely to spread or recur (reappear at some date following the original treatment).

Stage of cancer

We looked earlier at the clinical examination that a breast specialist will undertake when seeing a woman with breast cancer, and how extra tests can be used to determine how far the cancer may have spread at the time of the diagnosis. The extent of spread is the stage of the cancer.

When the pathologist has a tissue sample from a breast cancer to examine then he or she can also examine under the microscope the degree to which the cancer cells have spread away from their starting point. Cancer cells do this by pushing their way in between surrounding normal cells or by travelling along the lymph channels. Microscopic examination is of course able to show lymph spread at a very early stage, long before it shows as swollen lymph glands in clinical examination.

STAGING SYSTEMS

Specialists use internationally agreed systems of assessment and scoring to categorise breast cancer. This is useful to ensure that a woman's treatment is appropriate for the type of cancer she's got and that it takes account of how far it has already developed. It enables the results of research in one centre to be applied anywhere else, because there is a common language that different medical experts understand.

Two main classification systems are in use:

1 The 'TNM' (tumour, node, metastasis) system
2 The Stage I to IV system

1. The TNM system

In the TNM system a score is given to:

- T: the tumour according to its size and whether it is attached to the underlying chest wall
- N: to the nodes in the armpit or neck (i.e. whether they contain tumour cells)
- M: to the presence or absence of distant spread (metastases)

If, for example, a breast cancer is given a stage of $T_1N_0M_0$ this would mean a breast tumour less than 2cm in diameter, with no spread to lymph nodes and no metastases. $T_3N_3M_1$ means a tumour over 5cm in diameter plus lymph nodes in the neck plus distant spread.

2. The Stage system

This has four stages, is easier to understand and is also used in respect of breast cancer.

- *Stage 1* cancers are less than 2cm in diameter (as assessed on clinical examination). There are no cancer cells in the lymph glands in the armpit and there are no signs of the cancer anywhere else in the body.

- *Stage 2* cancers are between 2cm and 5cm in diameter. There may or may not be palpable swelling of the axillary lymph nodes but there is no apparent spread anywhere else in the body.
- *Stage 3* cancers are larger than 5cm diameter and there is palpable swelling of the lymph nodes in the axilla and/or at the neck, but no apparent spread anywhere else in the body.
- *Stage 4* cancers are of any size but the cancer has spread to parts of the body other than the lymph nodes.

Both the grade and the stage of breast cancer at diagnosis have a marked effect upon the outlook for the woman concerned. Women with grade 1 cells are twice as likely as those with grade 3 cells to survive another 10 years. Over 80 per cent of women at stage 1 when diagnosed are still alive five years later, but less than 20 per cent of those at stage 4 survive this long.

Non-invasive cancer

One of the main features that distinguish cancer cells from normal ones is their ability to invade other tissues. The cancers we've been referring to so far in this chapter are all invasive cancers.

However, in some types of breast disease some cancer-like changes occur but which do not necessarily lead on to breast cancer. The commonest of these is called 'ductal carcinoma in situ', or DCIS. ('Carcinoma' is an alternative word for cancer and 'in situ' refers to its staying put at the site of origin.) As the name suggests, DCIS originates from the duct cells. It only rarely causes a lump in the breast and is usually found as a result of screening mammograms, where it causes a characteristic speckled pattern to show up on the X-ray film. Over half of the women in whom DCIS is detected are past the menopause.

Exactly what happens to DCIS if it's left alone is uncertain, but a proportion of women with it do get invasive cancer in later years. It is not possible to predict which women with DCIS are at greater risk for developing breast cancer, nor is other information such as oestrogen receptor status any help. For this reason all women with DCIS are offered surgery to completely remove it. This is increasingly being done by means that preserve as much normal breast tissue as possible (see chapter 7) and may be combined with radiotherapy. The good news is that complete surgical removal of DCIS has nearly a 100 per cent success rate in preventing a later cancer developing. DCIS is therefore considered to be a *pre*-malignant type of breast change. It is not early breast cancer.

Lobular carcinoma in situ (LCIS) is a similar condition arising from the milk-producing lobes in the breast. It is less common than DCIS and tends to occur in pre-menopausal women. As it does not cause a palpable lump in the breast and does not show up on mammograms it is usually only discovered during the course of microscopic examination of breast tissue removed for another reason. LCIS probably does not turn into breast cancer but a woman who has it has a higher risk of developing breast cancer (in either breast) over the next several decades. It is therefore considered to be a risk factor for breast cancer rather than a pre-malignant condition.

Chapter 6

Overview of Treatment Options for Breast Cancer

No two women (or men) with breast cancer are exactly alike. In addition to the particular combination of tumour tissue type, grade and stage there are also general health factors to take into account, which may have an important bearing on what the treatment for any one individual should be. Breast cancer is an active area of medical research, so new treatments regularly come along or are being tested and existing treatments are continually being re-appraised for the best way in which to use them. There is therefore no standard way of treating breast cancer, which is one of the reasons why the treatment is now undertaken by specialist centres that have all the necessary skills in one place.

It's also important to point out that the treatment of breast cancer, as with any important disease, is not only about which drug or surgical technique to use, but also about taking care of the whole person. The emotional and social consequences of serious illness are seen in their sharpest focus in cancer. Excellent progress has also been made in this aspect of medical care in the past several years.

The goals of breast cancer treatment are therefore:

- to prevent the advance of the cancer or delay its recurrence for as long as possible
- to improve the quality of life for all patients, but especially those in whom 'cure' is not possible

As far as the cancer itself is concerned, there are four main groups of treatment available. They are not necessarily all applicable to everyone with breast cancer, and some of the circumstances in which one type is more appropriate than another will become clear later. In general the decision as to which treatment or combination of treatments is appropriate is decided on the basis of staging and pathology findings by a team consisting of all the relevant types of specialist in combination with the patient and her relatives or friends.

Surgery

Surgical removal of breast cancer has been and remains the mainstay of treatment, and most people with breast cancer will be offered surgery of one kind or another. Not very many years ago the commonest operation for breast cancer was the so-called 'radical mastectomy'. 'Mastectomy' means removal of the whole breast, and the 'radical' bit referred to the fact that the surgeon also took away all of the lymph nodes in the armpit plus the muscles underlying the breast in the belief that this gave the best chance of removing every cancerous cell. Such an extensive procedure is now hardly ever done and breast cancer surgery has evolved into a more subtle treatment in which the minimum amount of tissue is removed. The other techniques, such as X-rays and drug therapy that we'll cover shortly, allow the mopping up of stray cancer cells without the need for the aggressive surgery of old while at the same time actually achieving better results against the cancer.

Plastic surgery has produced methods to preserve or restore as much as possible the breast as part of a woman's body. Expertise in this area is also expanding, and the fact that cosmetically acceptable results can much more commonly be achieved means that less trauma is done to a woman's psychological health as well as her physical appearance.

TUMOUR REMOVAL

In general, a small breast cancer is completely removed along with a 1cm margin of normal breast tissue – this is called wide local excision, WLE or 'lumpectomy' and is usually done under general anaesthetic. When the cancer is large, or is scattered through a wide area of the breast or indeed if there is more than one area in the breast that has turned cancerous, as does sometimes happen, then the whole breast may still need to be removed, but nowadays the muscles beneath the breast are left intact.

The more conservative surgical procedures (wide local excision) are usually combined with radiotherapy (see below) whereas sometimes more extensive surgery does not need to be. As always, much depends on individual circumstance so one can only talk in general terms here.

LYMPH NODE REMOVAL

Part of the logic that guided surgeons 20 years ago to take away the lymph nodes in the armpit was that by doing so they were removing cancer cells that had already spread there, even if they were not obvious. Secondly, by removing the nodes one reduced the chance of the cancer later re-appearing within the axillary lymph nodes where it could give rise to other problems such as blockage of the lymph drainage of the arm. These were reasonable assumptions but there were problems in practice.

First was the observation that the long-term survival of women who had the more radical surgery was no better than those who just had the lump removed and not the whole breast. We now realise that spread of breast cancer actually occurs much earlier than previously thought, so many of the women had radical surgery in vain – the tumour was already out and away. Secondly, the deliberate removal of all the lymph nodes severely interrupted the drainage of lymph from the arm as a direct result of the surgery. So this potential complication that might have been many years down the line was occurring more or less right away, which was a major disadvantage of that approach.

There is still an ongoing debate about the value of lymph node removal and how to do it with the least amount of trouble to the patient. Knowing that there has been spread to the lymph nodes has a significant impact on the woman's outlook but if that were the only benefit then it couldn't be justified as a procedure. However, knowledge of the lymph node status can make a difference to the choice of treatment appropriate for an individual person, so the information is valuable and the procedure is still regularly done.

Effective compromises that allow the necessary information to be gained with the minimum degree of side effects are the techniques of:

- *lymph node sampling*, where four representative lymph nodes are removed

- *sentinel node biopsy,* where the first (sentinel) lymph node that cancer cells might spread to is identified using blue dye injected into the lymph vessels and a weakly radioactive tracer material. If the sentinel node does not contain any cancer cells then the conclusion is that spread has not yet occurred and no further lymph nodes need be removed. The results of several large research studies investigating the modern role of axillary node removal and sentinel node biopsy are awaited and will clear up this uncertainty.

BREAST RECONSTRUCTION
This is covered in more detail in chapter 7.

Radiotherapy

Radiotherapy is the use of radiation to kill cancer cells. The principle behind using X-rays is that the high level of energy they have is able to damage the DNA inside cells and therefore disrupts the ability of cells to divide and multiply. Because cancer cells reproduce at a much faster rate than normal cells they are more vulnerable to X-rays, but some damage to normal tissue is unavoidable in radiotherapy. Because of the position of the breast on the front of the chest wall it is however easier to deliver X-rays to breast tissue with minimal damage to other normal tissues than it is for cancers deep within the body. The heart is the most important structure that is sufficiently near to the breasts to be possibly in the line of fire but this is much less of a problem with modern equipment, in which the X-ray beam can be very well focussed.

Sometimes radiotherapy is used prior to surgery to help reduce the size of a large cancer of the breast but usually it is used several weeks following surgery, when the wounds have well healed. The treatment is given to the breast region from which the cancer was removed, possibly also to the armpit in order to kill off cancer cells in the remaining lymph nodes and an extra dose is given to the operation scar after lumpectomy to deal with any cancer cells that might be present there.

RADIOTHERAPY IN PRACTICE

A radiotherapy session is quite brief, just a few minutes long, but needs to be repeated. A typical course would be every day Monday to Friday for five to six weeks but there are research studies currently in process to compare different schedules for their relative benefits. The first radiotherapy session is longer to allow the radiotherapist to set up the machine accurately against the exact position of the woman's chest wall. Pen marks aid the setting up process in later sessions and, with the woman's permission, a tiny permanent tattoo acts as an accurate reference mark.

Although modern radiotherapy is well tolerated it can have some side effects. Tiredness is quite common. Skin irritation, which is like sunburn, can occur and proper skin care is important. Generally this includes being very careful with washing and drying and avoiding skin creams and deodorants until it settles, which can take some weeks after the radiotherapy course is complete. Extremes of temperature, such as from hot water bottles or ice packs, should be temporarily avoided, as should sunlight exposure.

Other possible side effects include a cough and dryness of the throat on swallowing which tend to happen at about the third week of treatment and which also can persist for a while. The treated breast can feel rather heavy and if treatment is given to the nodes in the armpit then arm swelling can occur due to the accumulation of lymph (lymphoedema). Radiotherapy staff are very experienced in the practical management of all of these problems and can offer helpful advice.

The main benefit of radiotherapy is that it reduces the likelihood of cancer recurring at the original site and it does improve the long-term survival rates from breast cancer. Presently under study is the use of special X-ray machines that can deliver a very localised X-ray beam that can be used during the operation. This targets the cancerous area very accurately and with minimal side effects.

Chemotherapy

The use of drugs to kill cancer cells is called chemotherapy. Generally speaking cancer drugs work along similar lines to radiotherapy because they target the cell's 'machinery' for the duplication of DNA. As with radiotherapy, cancer drugs are not completely selective and they can damage normal cells too. The bone marrow is where we manufacture new blood cells continuously and it is particularly vulnerable to the effects of chemotherapy. This is why regular blood checks are a normal part of the routine when receiving chemotherapy. Hair, fingernails and the lining cells of the digestive system are other parts of the body with a naturally high rate of production of new cells, so hair loss, mouth ulcers and digestive upset can be side effects too. Fatigue can be prominent.

Modern chemotherapy treatments are much better tolerated than older regimes and we now have effective medicines to combat nausea and other side effects but it can't be denied that chemotherapy can be hard going at times. Fortunately the worst spells are brief and not everyone experiences them.

CHEMOTHERAPY IN PRACTICE
The majority of people receive chemotherapy as an outpatient procedure in a unit specifically set up for the purpose and run by specially trained nurses and doctors. These are usually pretty busy places.

Some drugs are taken by mouth but most are given through a drip set up in a vein. Following a general check-over including a blood test to ensure that the bone marrow has recovered following the last session of treatment the drugs are given over a period of a few hours. Typically six episodes of treatment are given, spaced at three to four week intervals. By combining different drugs better results are obtained than with one alone.

Although the bone marrow is given time to recover between treatment sessions there will usually be some drop in the production of new red blood cells during the course. Red blood cells carry oxygen and a lack of them is what causes anaemia, which is one of the reasons for the fatigue that accompanies chemotherapy. The white cells of our blood are also made in the bone marrow and their production also falls due to chemotherapy. As we rely on our white cells to fight infection, people on chemotherapy are more vulnerable to catching infections. It's therefore important to try and avoid contact with people who have heavy colds or other easily spread infections, and to report symptoms such as a sore throat or a temperature to a doctor right away. The low point in a person's blood cell counts is usually about seven to 10 days following the chemotherapy, so that's the time to be most vigilant.

Hair loss occurs with most chemotherapy but the extent varies between the different drugs in use. It recovers fully after the treatment is over and breast cancer care centres can provide good quality wigs in the interim.

RESEARCH TRIALS

The details of the drugs in use are complex but some examples are listed below. New combinations are almost always being tested under research conditions. Most patients with breast cancer will find that their regional treatment centre will be involved in one or more such studies and this may mean that they will be offered the opportunity to join one. If so the details will always be fully explained. The final decision about entering a research trial always rests with the patient.

EXAMPLES OF CHEMOTHERAPY DRUGS USED IN TREATING BREAST CANCER

Some of the most useful anti-cancer drugs have been around for many years. Cyclophosphamide for example is a 'nitrogen mustard' and related to the 'mustard gas' used in the First World War. Cyclophosphamide forms a bond between the two strands of the DNA molecule, preventing it from unzipping, which is an essential requirement when a cell reproduces. Cyclophosphamide is combined with two drugs that interfere with the ability of cells to make DNA (methotrexate and fluorouracil) in one of the main drug combinations used against breast cancer (commonly referred to as 'CMF'). Another combination is of cyclophosphamide with doxorubicin, a drug that seizes up the process of DNA duplication. One of the main limiting factors with doxorubicin is that it can damage heart muscle. This restricts the total dose that can be safely given and may make it unsuitable for use in people who already have heart disease. It also causes more hair loss than some other drugs.

Plants have been the source of some of the most powerful anti-cancer drugs and the taxanes are a group of drugs derived from the yew tree. Docetaxel and paclitaxel are taxanes used for advanced breast cancer where earlier chemotherapy has failed but they are also being investigated for use in early breast cancer.

REDUCING THE SIDE EFFECTS OF CHEMOTHERAPY

- Nausea and vomiting can be caused by chemotherapy because of a direct action of the drugs on an area within the brain that controls vomiting. Granisetron and ondansetron are drugs that block this happening, so these problems are much less common than they used to be.
- Hair loss can be reduced by techniques to cool the scalp during chemotherapy sessions. By dropping the temperature of the hair roots their metabolism is reduced, which lowers their tendency to take up the chemotherapy drugs from the bloodstream.
- Excessive fall in the blood count caused by chemotherapy may cause a delay before the next session can safely be given. However, too much delay may reduce the effectiveness of the chemotherapy against the breast cancer. In some patients it may therefore be necessary to use a hormone capable of stimulating the bone marrow to recover more quickly between chemotherapy sessions.
- The commonest side effect, fatigue, is the hardest to help with drugs. Support from family, friends, caring agencies and all of the health professionals is needed at this time.

TIMING OF CHEMOTHERAPY

Chemotherapy has usually been used following surgery for the cancer with the aim of dealing with any abnormal cells that have spread elsewhere in the body. It can also be used prior to surgery to help reduce the size of a breast cancer and so make the operation easier. Much research is still going on to establish the best way to time the use of chemotherapy and combine it with all the other methods of tackling breast cancer.

Hormone therapies

We've already noted that some breast cancers are sensitive to oestrogen, and that by removing oestrogen or blocking its effect we can turn off stimulation to the breast cancer cells. The two ways in which this can be achieved are:

1 Remove or 'shut down' the ovaries, thus switching off the production of oestrogen. The medical term for this is 'ovarian ablation'.
2 Use drug therapy to block the effects of oestrogen.

1. REMOVAL OR 'SWITCHING OFF' THE OVARIES

There are several ways of achieving this:

Surgery

Surgical removal of the ovaries is a fairly straightforward procedure that can be done with 'keyhole' surgery techniques. It involves a general anaesthetic and some small surgical incisions on the tummy, through which the instruments are placed.

X-rays

Exposing the ovaries to carefully targeted X-rays permanently stops them producing any more hormones. The effect is the same as removing them surgically, but avoids an operation. Although modern X-ray treatment is very accurate it is impossible to achieve an adequate dose of X-rays to the ovaries and at the same time completely avoid damage to surrounding tissues. The bowel and the bladder are close by and so one can get diarrhoea or bladder irritation, which can last some weeks after the X-ray treatment.

Drug therapy

Surgery or X-rays to the ovaries cause permanent sterility. For a younger woman with breast cancer who plans to have more children eventually they may therefore be unsuitable. One possible option is to use a medicine called goserelin, which is a synthetic version of a hormone naturally released by the brain and which normally is involved in the control of ovarian function. When goserelin is given continuously it causes the ovaries to cease production of oestrogen and progesterone. If goserelin is stopped then the ovaries slowly regain function, so fertility is regained. As you might expect the practicalities of using goserelin are not quite so straightforward, but the impact of treatment on fertility is an area that the breast cancer specialist can fully discuss with a woman in relation to her own circumstances.

Ovarian ablation is only of use when the ovaries are still working: there is no point in this treatment in women who develop breast cancer following the menopause. In practice, therefore, it is used only in women under 50 years old

2. DRUGS THAT BLOCK THE EFFECTS OF OESTROGEN

Tamoxifen

Tamoxifen has probably been the most important of all breast cancer drugs over the past 20 years. It is an anti-oestrogen, which means it blocks the effect of oestrogen circulating round the blood from latching on to target tissues. It is taken as a tablet once a day. It is only useful in women who have ER +ve breast cancer, in whom it significantly reduces their death rate. Tamoxifen very slightly increases the risks of developing cancer of the lining of the womb and of developing clots in the veins, but the potential advantages of the drug considerably outweigh the disadvantages in the treatment of breast cancer.

Tamoxifen is useful in women with breast cancer both before and after the menopause. This is because in post-menopausal women, although the ovaries have shut down, the small amount of oestrogen that continues to be made by fatty tissue is enough to continue stimulating ER +ve breast cancer cells.

Drugs that block oestrogen production – the 'aromatase inhibitors'

Almost every chemical reaction of importance in the body is helped to take place by the action of an enzyme. Enzymes are proteins with custom-designed shapes, each one specific for a particular reaction. Enzymes work in various ways but the commonest is because their shape brings together more easily the various substances that are combined in the chemical process they are involved in.

The important enzyme in the production of oestrogen by the ovaries and by fatty tissue elsewhere is called aromatase. We now have several drugs that are capable of blocking the action of aromatase, which therefore causes oestrogen production to fall. Anastrozole is the best known of these 'aromatase inhibitors'. The others in use are letrozole and exemestane. Several studies have shown these drugs to be effective in treating breast cancer and more research is ongoing to determine how best to combine them with the other available treatments to get the best results.

There may also be additional benefits from the aromatase inhibitors. For example, they do not increase the chance of clots occurring in the veins.

Combination therapy

The various treatments for breast cancer are used together to maximise their effect. Surgery to remove a breast cancer is generally combined with radiotherapy, and followed up with chemotherapy. Ovarian ablation may be added for pre-menopausal women. The number of potential combinations is large but for each woman there will be a smaller range of choices that suit her own circumstances and the breast cancer team are there to provide the necessary expert advice.

Some women are keen to be fully informed of all possible options and will take an active role in deciding what treatment to have. Others feel most comfortable with delegating the decision making entirely to the breast cancer team. All need to have confidence in the expertise and commitment of the professionals involved in their care. Despite the media stories that occasionally reveal the unsurprising truth that no system is perfect, including the National Health Service, a woman with breast cancer receiving treatment in the UK can be confident that she is being treated to a standard that is the equal of the best in any other country in the world.

The main tools at the disposal of the breast cancer team are therefore surgery, radiotherapy, chemotherapy and hormone treatment. The two situations in which these treatments are used are:

1 The treatment of the breast cancer when it is first diagnosed (called the primary cancer).
2 The treatment of recurrent cancer some time after primary treatment.

These are the situations that we'll now cover in more detail.

Chapter 7

Treatment of Primary Breast Cancer

The main aims of treating breast cancer when it first appears (primary breast cancer) are to:

- remove or destroy the cancer as much as is feasible and necessary
- minimise the cosmetic effects of treatment
- reduce the long term likelihood of recurrence of the cancer

Surgical removal of the breast cancer was the original method of treatment and is still the mainstay. Radiotherapy is the other main method of dealing with the cancer at its site of origin. One can call these 'local treatments'. In the majority of women local treatments will be combined with others to deal with cancer cells that have spread away from the original source. This is because we now better understand the behaviour of breast cancer cells and how they interact with the rest of the body.

Breast cancer behaviour

One of the main advances in the understanding of breast cancer has been that it behaves differently to what might be called the classic cancer model. In this model a tumour grows in the original spot until it gets to a certain size and then after some time spreads in a more or less predictable way to the local lymph glands and then, usually much later, it spreads further throughout the body (metastasises). Many cancers do follow this pattern – cancer of the bowel (colon) being a good example.

However, analysis of the outcome of women who had operable breast cancers removed along with radiotherapy to the local lymph nodes showed that a proportion of them still ultimately developed metastases. The conclusion had to be that breast cancer spread early and that microscopic metastases were already present in a high proportion of women at the time of diagnosis. This applied even when these women had gone to their doctor without delay after noticing the symptoms of breast cancer and had been treated quickly thereafter.

Treatment strategies therefore changed to take this into account, and so was developed the concept of 'adjuvant' treatment.

Adjuvant treatment

'Adjuvant' is an adjective that means 'assisting' or 'helping another' and is used in breast cancer to mean the use of extra treatments right from the start. So not only does the surgeon remove the tumour if at all feasible and follows this up with radiotherapy to control the disease at the site of origin and first likely point of spread to the armpit (i.e. local treatment) but also adjuvant chemotherapy and hormone treatments may be introduced at this stage too. In earlier methods of treatment the tumour removal, along with radiotherapy would have been the standard first-line treatment and the other types of therapy would only have been brought in some time later, if there were signs of the cancer 'coming back'.

Now adjuvant therapy is given on the assumption that the tumour needs to be treated *as if* it has already spread at the time of first diagnosis. Until fairly recently the sequence would have been surgery first, then other treatments. Now adjuvant therapy is increasingly being used prior to surgery when it is called neoadjuvant therapy, with the aim of reducing tumour size and making the operation less extensive (e.g. a wide local excision rather than a mastectomy), involving less loss of breast tissue.

Combination treatment

The subject of which type of adjuvant treatment to choose for an individual person is too complex to cover in detail, and in any case is very much an individualised decision. But generally speaking:

- Pre-menopausal women who have ER +ve cancers are offered treatment to remove or shut down the ovaries.
- Tamoxifen is usually offered to all women with ER +ve breast cancer (irrespective of age) for up to five years. The aromatase inhibitors (anastrozole, letrozole, exemestane) may be used alternatively in post-menopausal women.
- Chemotherapy is more likely to be helpful in women below 60 years old, who have a large tumour, who have spread of the cancer to the local lymph nodes or who have ER -ve breast cancer.
- Chemotherapy can be given first and then the woman can take

tamoxifen. (Tamoxifen is not given at the same time as chemo-therapy as it reduces its effectiveness.)

Types of breast surgery

The simplest breast lump removal involves the tumour itself plus a 1cm margin of surrounding healthy breast tissue. This is the 'lumpectomy' mentioned in the previous chapter. Among the many factors that determine whether a lumpectomy is sufficient treatment is the woman's own feelings about whether she is confident to have a limited amount of breast tissue removed. Some women feel more secure if the whole breast is removed. This is obviously a personal decision that needs to be made in conjunction with the breast cancer team.

MASTECTOMY

When it is necessary to remove the breast there are several surgical ways of doing so. Sometimes the breast tissue can be removed while leaving the skin and the nipple intact. This allows the breast to be reconstructed right away, usually using an artifical implant under the skin to fill out the breast shape. The obvious benefit of such a procedure is that there is an immediate good cosmetic result. The technique is not suitable for all types of breast cancer but is more often used when ductal carcinoma in situ (DCIS) is detected on mammogram and is the only condition needing treatment.

In so-called 'simple mastectomy' the whole breast, including the nipple, is removed. A 'modified radical mastectomy' is the same plus the removal of a limited amount of underlying muscle. This is combined with removal of lymph nodes from the axilla and, as was mentioned in chapter 6, a 'sentinel node' biopsy may be used to determine whether it is necessary to remove more of the lymph nodes.

Breast reconstruction

The techniques available to produce a good cosmetic result are improving and an increasing proportion of women who have had breast surgery will go on to have treatment to restore the appearance of their breast as much as possible.

The techniques include:

SILICONE GEL IMPLANTS

Despite the bad press that silicone gel implants have had, especially in the USA, it is still the belief of medical experts in the UK that they are completely safe. If a woman's natural breasts are fairly small then it may be possible to insert an adequately sized gel implant at the time of the first surgery. For those women with larger breasts a tissue expander can be inserted which can be gradually inflated over a period of some months. This stretches the skin overlying the breast so that it can accommodate a larger gel implant at a later operation. Further techniques are now used which include inflatable implants that have a valve that does not need to be removed once the implant is up to an adequate size. This makes a second implant operation unnecessary (see figure 4).

SKIN AND MUSCLE FLAPS

Different techniques may be needed when larger amounts of skin and tissue have to be removed during the primary surgery. This may not leave enough skin to be suitable for stretching over an implant. Also, radiotherapy following surgery can affect the overlying skin such that it may not respond well to skin stretching techniques. In those circumstances the skills of the plastic surgeon are required.

Figure 4: Breast reconstruction technique using tissue expansion

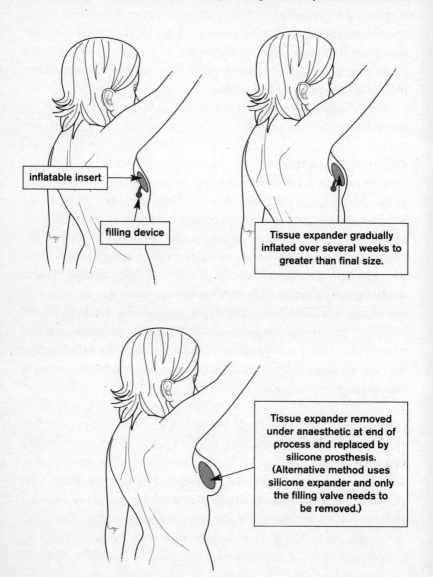

inflatable insert

filling device

Tissue expander gradually inflated over several weeks to greater than final size.

Tissue expander removed under anaesthetic at end of process and replaced by silicone prosthesis. (Alternative method uses silicone expander and only the filling valve needs to be removed.)

One of the many techniques that have been developed by plastic surgeons over decades has been the transplanting of skin and underlying tissue from one part of the body to another. Provided one does this carefully so that the blood supply to the part being moved is maintained, it can be very successful. To do this the area to be moved is detached most of the way round, keeping a stalk of tissue attached, through which blood can reach the movable area. The surgeon then closes over the 'donor area', which heals like any operation. This does mean that there is a scar at the donor site, but it is out of the way and can easily be concealed by clothing. The movable area can then be swung into position where it is required. In the case of a breast cancer operation this is of course to the defect in the breast caused by the removal of the cancer.

In the case of breast cancer two techniques of this type are in common use. The first uses a donor area below the shoulder blade on the same side as the breast cancer. This 'flap' technique is named after the muscle involved, which is called *latissimus dorsi*.

Alternatively a similar flap can be made from the front of the abdomen and swung upwards or transplanted to the breast area. The muscle of the front of the abdomen is called *rectus abdominis*, so this flap is called the TRAM flap (transverse rectus abdominis myocutaneous: myo=muscle, cutaneous=skin). More recently, the amount of muscle being removed has been minimised by relying on smaller blood vessels to supply the flap. This is known by the anatomical name of these blood vessels and is called the DIEP flap (Deep Inferior Epigastric Pedicle).

Because such transplants use the patient's own tissue, there is no problem with rejection such as occurs in transplants between different people (see figure 5).

Figure 5: 'TRAM' and 'latissimus dorsi' flaps for breast reconstruction

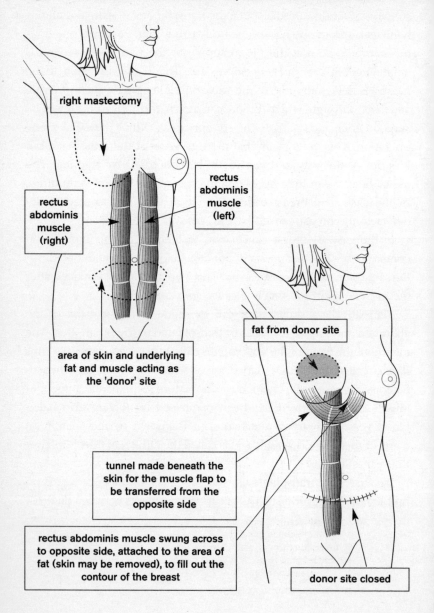

right mastectomy

rectus abdominis muscle (left)

rectus abdominis muscle (right)

area of skin and underlying fat and muscle acting as the 'donor' site

fat from donor site

tunnel made beneath the skin for the muscle flap to be transferred from the opposite side

rectus abdominis muscle swung across to opposite side, attached to the area of fat (skin may be removed), to fill out the contour of the breast

donor site closed

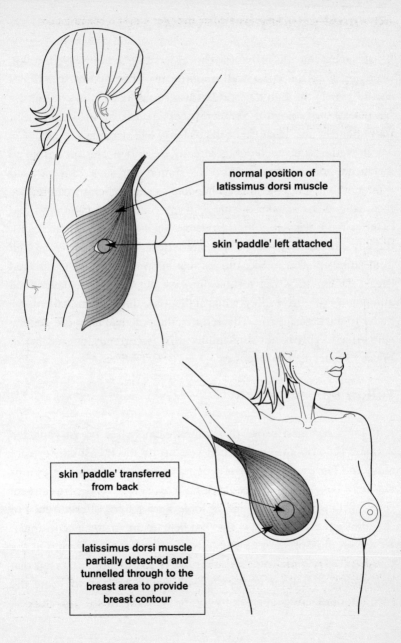

normal position of
latissimus dorsi muscle

skin 'paddle' left attached

skin 'paddle' transferred
from back

latissimus dorsi muscle
partially detached and
tunnelled through to the
breast area to provide
breast contour

Advanced primary breast cancer

What is meant by this is that the cancer has spread to involve the skin overlying it or the chest wall underneath it but otherwise has not spread widely through the body. Advanced primary cancer can arise because of the biological peculiarities of a particular breast cancer, or unfortunately also because of neglect and late diagnosis.

All of the same techniques already described are applicable to advanced primary cancer. Whereas surgery for such cancers used often not to be possible, this is changing as chemotherapy can reduce the size and the activity of such cancers (neoadjuvant therapy) and make surgery feasible. One of the potential ways in which chemotherapy can be used with fewer side effects is to deliver it through guide tubes placed in the arteries that supply blood to the affected breast. Doing so is not technically easy but allows a smaller total amount of drugs to be used while at the same time targeting the drugs better to the breast tissue. This reduces the potential for more general side effects. This is not a technique that is currently offered by all breast cancer treatment centres.

Follow up

It follows common sense that after treatment for breast cancer a woman will continue to be followed up by the breast cancer care team and her own GP, the aims being to answer ongoing questions she may have, to look out for long-term side effects of treatment (e.g. swelling of the arm) and to look out for signs of recurrence of the tumour and so allow the medical team to act accordingly. However, the optimum timetable for follow up is not clear. On the one hand very widely spaced intervals of follow up may mean that any recurrent tumour is already well established by the time the next appointment occurs. But very frequent follow up runs the risk of creating an unhelpful degree of anxiety in the woman and her family.

PROS AND CONS OF FOLLOW UP

Detecting recurrence of cancer early does not automatically mean that further treatment will be possible or any more effective than if it is delayed a while longer. One could argue that early detection of recurrence merely extends the time that a woman is aware that her cancer has reappeared, without changing the ultimate outcome, which is a dubious benefit. Striking a reasonable balance ensures adequately close monitoring for signs of recurrent breast cancer at the site of the operation, which often can be helped by further treatment. This might be surgery, radiotherapy (if it was not used in the primary treatment), chemotherapy, hormone treatment or bisphosphonate therapy (see later).

There are additional benefits from reasonably frequent follow up, not least of which is the help and support from the health team in coping with the cancer and dealing with the practical issues that arise.

FREQUENCY AND NATURE OF FOLLOW UP

Although the exact details will vary, follow up of women after their first treatment for breast cancer will typically be every six months for two years and then annually thereafter. However, the nurses in the breast care team can handle queries at any time. If chemotherapy is being used then more frequent follow up by the chemotherapy expert (oncologist) will be usual until the treatment is complete. Because of the multi-professional nature of modern breast cancer treatment there are often combined clinics at which the various health professionals come together and co-ordinate their input for each individual patient.

Also the exact nature of the follow up will vary. Clinical examination, inspection of the surgical site, feeling for enlargement of the lymph nodes under the armpit and at the neck, and simple blood tests are routine and carried out on almost everyone. Mammography may or may not be needed or be helpful on the side of the treated breast as the treatment itself may make it hard to detect or assess any further changes. However, there is a need to keep a close watch on the opposite breast as there is a higher risk of cancer developing in the opposite breast in women who have had breast cancer.

Chapter 8

Treatment of Advanced (Metastatic) Breast Cancer

By 'advanced' breast cancer we mean here cancer that has spread away from the primary site to more distant parts of the body. This is more correctly called metastatic breast cancer.

As we mentioned in the last chapter, breast cancer treatment is now geared to the idea that it can spread quite early on in its course of development, hence the use of adjuvant treatment. It will hopefully by now also be clear that breast cancer is not one disease, but many. Some of the differences between breast cancers, such as hormone receptor status, we are beginning to understand and can take account of in treatment. Other differences are as yet beyond our understanding and account for much of the unpredictability that accompanies breast cancer.

Ultimately breast cancer is still a disease that has a high chance of spreading to other parts of the body, even though this may be many years after the primary illness. When such metastases appear it has a significant impact on a woman's outlook. Although there is quite a large margin either side, the average length of time a woman will survive after the development of metastatic breast cancer is about two years although this time scale is increasing with modern treatments.

Developments in the treatment of metastatic cancer are showing much promise but the reality is that 'cure' is not an aim of treatment of advanced breast cancer. Realistic goals need to be set, and are far more likely to be achieved, as a result. Good treatment of metastatic cancer, of breast as well as of any other tissue, is focussed on:

- symptom control
- extending survival when reasonably possible
- respecting the patient's wishes

This is not intended as an order of priority, and modern health care places patients in the centre of the decision-making process, if that's where they want to be. Much of the 'fear' that still attaches to cancer is because of a lack of awareness of just how good modern cancer management has become. The limelight, perhaps inevitably, tends to be stolen by 'cancer-beating drugs' that offer a chance of 'cure'. Yet we know that none of us is immortal and that cancer is but one of the many possible reasons why we all eventually die. So although advanced or metastatic breast cancer carries with it, generally speaking, a much foreshortened life expectancy what we must concentrate on is ensuring that the *quality* of a person's remaining life is made as good as it can be.

Sites of spread of breast cancer

The problems that arise from metastatic breast cancer arise mostly as a direct result of the region in the body where the cancer cells settle. Bone is the commonest site of spread, perhaps because of the meshwork structure within bones, which may trap and hold cancer cells circulating in the blood more easily than other tissues. The lungs, liver and brain are the other main sites about which some general comments can be made.

BONES

Bones are active parts of the body, continuously in a state of repair and remodelling. There are two main groups of cells within bone, one of which, in effect, breaks bone down into its component minerals, and the other group of cells refashions new bone. This seemingly pointless activity is quite the reverse as it makes it possible for bone to adapt to change. Thus after a fracture occurs in normal bone the bone-building cells go into overdrive. Less dramatically, increased bone-building activity allows bone to thicken up in areas of increased loading.

Bisphosphonates

Bisphosphonates are drugs that slow the rate at which bone is dissolved, thus favouring a build-up in bone strength over time. The main use of bisphosphonates is to help prevent the weakening of bones that occurs in older people, particularly in women, and which has nothing to do with cancer (osteoporosis). However, they appear to also help prevent the weakening of bone that can occur when cancer cells spread to the bones.

Bone pain and fractures

A cancer 'deposit' within the bones can give rise to pain, or can weaken the bone structure. A weakened bone, especially if within the weight-bearing parts of the skeleton such as the spine or the femur (thigh bone), may result in a breakage or crumbling of the bone at that point. When a bone breaks at the site of a cancer cell deposit it is called a 'pathological fracture'. Pathological fractures can be difficult to treat and they do not repair themselves like ordinary bone. Treatment of a fracture in an important bone such as the femur will require the insertion of a metal pin to give the region extra strength, and then be followed with radiotherapy to destroy the cancer cells at the site. Radiotherapy to bony metastases can also be remarkably effective in reducing bone pain.

Predicting whether a pathological fracture may occur in advance, based on the evidence of X-rays and bone scans, and perhaps symptoms such as rapidly increasing localised pain is an inexact science. Sometimes, though, the risk of a fracture occurring is judged to be high enough to warrant advance treatment with an operation to attach or insert strengthening metal pins through the affected area of bone, followed by radiotherapy.

Non-steroidal anti-inflammatory drugs ('NSAIDs', such as ibuprofen, diclofenac) are also commonly very helpful at reducing the amount of bone pain caused by metastatic cancer.

Radiotherapy is only practical for small regions of bone affected by cancer spread. If there is a widespread distribution of cancer cells throughout the bones it becomes impractical to use radiotherapy. Chemotherapy and hormone treatments, much as already described for primary breast cancer may be used in those circumstances.

Anaemia

As the bone marrow is the site of manufacture of new blood cells extensive replacement of the bone marrow by tumour cells can give rise to anaemia. In older patients unfit for too much in the way of chemotherapy it may be best to simply use a blood transfusion every now and again to 'top up' the level of circulating blood cells and thus counteract the anaemia.

Calcium

The level of calcium in the blood is normally controlled within quite narrow limits by the complex interacting effects of vitamin D and hormones upon the bones (the main store of calcium) and the kidneys, liver, skin and digestive system. One of the effects cancer can have when it spreads to the bones is to cause an excess of calcium to leak into the blood. A raised level of calcium in the blood is called hypercalcaemia. Mild hypercalcaemia causes thirst and the passage of excess amounts of urine. As calcium levels climb so the effects become more serious, including tiredness, nausea, vomiting, constipation, drowsiness and confusion. This can happen over quite a short period of time in the case of metastatic bone disease. Treatment in the form of intravenous drips providing extra fluids help to flush out the excess calcium and the bisphosphonate drugs given into a drip can cause a rapid lowering of the calcium, which will remain so for a few weeks. It's important for the doctor to remember to check the blood calcium level regularly in patients who have metastatic bone disease in order to pick this up.

LUNGS

In normal health each lung completely fills its space in the cavity within each side of the chest. The lungs are covered in a thin lubricated membrane, called the pleura (pronounced *'ploo-rah'*), which aids their movement during breathing. In advanced breast cancer some cancer cells can reach the pleura, leading to a marked increase in the amount of fluid produced. This fluid, which is called a pleural effusion, partially occupies the space intended for the lungs so it can cause breathlessness. Removing some of the fluid is quite an easy procedure that can be done under local anaesthetic, and doing so makes it easier to breathe. However, the fluid tends to re-accumulate. To reduce the chance of this happening an anti-cancer drug can be injected into the fluid. If that fails then talcum powder injected instead will cause an inflammatory reaction that results in the pleura sticking to the inside of the chest cavity, which helps resist the re-accumulation of the fluid.

LIVER

Like the bones, the liver is a common site of spread of cancer cells. The normal liver has a great many tasks to carry out. It is the main site of the storage form of glucose (sugar) that we need between meals to keep us supplied with energy and it takes part in many hundreds of chemical reactions that help to cleanse the blood and eliminate waste products through the bile. Fortunately the liver has a large amount of spare capacity, so even when tests show that a lot of the liver is occupied by metastatic cancer this does not always mean that the patient feels particularly unwell. Although some limited success has been had with techniques to deliver chemotherapy to local areas within the liver affected by single clusters of cancer cells the more common situation is that liver metastases are multiple, and such treatments are impracticable and ineffective. High doses of steroid tablets (called dexamethasone) can be used to 'shrink' the liver, which can be useful if the liver is being stretched by the presence of the tumour cells within it, leading to pain. Extensive involvement of the liver with tumour cells indicates advanced cancer and a poor outlook for survival thereafter.

BRAIN

Spread of cancer cells to the brain is a very poor sign and patients in whom this has occurred will generally not survive for more than a few more months. The skull is fixed in volume, so tumour cells compress normal brain tissue and can therefore lead to a host of problems including confusion, loss of power and co-ordination, fits and other abnormalities of the nervous system. High dose steroids (dexamethasone) can shrink the tumour (or tumours, as they are often multiple), which can give temporary improvement. Radiotherapy can sometimes also be used for symptom relief, but it does not improve survival.

Types of treatment

These are similar to those used in treating primary breast cancer:

- *Hormone treatments*. In women with oestrogen receptor positive cancer, ovarian ablation and anti-oestrogen drugs such as tamoxifen in pre-menopausal women and tamoxifen and aromatase inhibitors in post-menopausal women.
- *Chemotherapy*. Including familiar combinations such as 'CMF' (page 65) and newer drugs such as the taxanes (page 65). Vinorelbine is an option for patients in whom prior treatment with drugs such as doxorubicin has failed to control the disease. Chemotherapy remains the preferred treatment in pre and post-menopausal women who have ER -ve breast cancer.
- *Radiotherapy*. Radiotherapy can be useful both in controlling metastases such as those described in bone, or in controlling recurrence of the cancer at the original site. Practical considerations, such as whether there has been previous radiotherapy to the same area, may limit the dose that can be safely tolerated by the skin and surrounding tissues in later sessions.

- *Newer treatments*. Bisphosphonates can be particularly useful to treat bone metastases. Trastuzumab is an antibody active against breast cancer cells found to produce an excess of certain proteins such as the HER-2 protein (page 44).

Drug costs and availability

Among the issues that are under scrutiny concerning all drugs, but particularly many of the anti-cancer drugs, are their costs. Many are very expensive, more so the newer drugs, about which we have insufficient knowledge yet of their usefulness and activity. Drug funding and availability is an emotive issue for a host of reasons. Media channels love to publish feel-good stories about the latest wonder medicine long before it is clear what the benefits and dangers of it are in the real world. The delivery of cancer services, although generally high in the UK, is not always faultlessly organised and can lead to much frustration on the part of patient and carers alike. The organisation of funding within the NHS is far from properly sorted out and the problem of 'postcode prescribing', in which treatments funded in one area may not be in another, although ethically unacceptable, persists.

The National Institute for Clinical Excellence (NICE) is a government-funded body set up to advise on the appropriate way in which medicines will be made available under the NHS and NICE has produced guidelines covering many of the drugs involved in the care of patients with breast cancer. In the main these are helpful and follow the best available medical knowledge so that patients with breast cancer can expect to receive such drugs when it is appropriate for their care, no matter where it is that they stay in the UK. Such is only as it should be, but it remains a distant goal for many of the areas in medicine that are as deserving of attention as breast cancer. NICE has many critics but at least we have a system in the UK that is actively engaged in trying to appraise the appropriate use of these drugs and provide clear guidance on how to use them.

Drug Trials

There are numerous research studies (also known as trials) going on in breast cancer and most if not all breast cancer treatment centres in the UK are likely to be involved in such research. This means that there is a fair chance that you will be offered the opportunity to take part in such a study. Doing so does of course advance medical knowledge in the only way that is truly helpful, which is to discover what works in people and not just in the laboratories, but such studies can take years to run their course and deliver results. Even so those results may not prove that the new treatment is any better than the old.

If a treatment exists which is known to be effective, then the structure of a modern research study will be to compare the new treatment against the old one. It will not be to compare the new treatment against no treatment at all, as to do so would be unethical. Patients need to be offered at least the best that we currently have available. Many patients feel happy to be part of a research trial. Often it is the only realistic way to get treatment that is thought to be an advance on the best currently in use. However, participation in a research trial must always be done according to strict rules concerning its appropriateness for the individual concerned. They are always designed so that you can withdraw for any reason at any time.

Many trials test one or more anti-cancer drugs against each other but there are trials that test different ways of giving radiotherapy or alternative surgical approaches. It is because of such surgical trials that we can now advise a woman with a small breast cancer that she can be treated by wide local excision and radiotherapy rather than to have to undergo a mastectomy.

Chapter 9

Male Breast Cancer

Cancer of the male breast is rare, comprising less than 1 per cent of all male cancers. The grades and stages of breast cancer that occur in males are much the same as for female breast cancer. Unfortunately male breast cancers tend to be more advanced by the time of diagnosis, partly because the cancer can erode through the skin at a smaller size but also because of a lack of awareness that male breast cancer exists. They tend to occur in older men and often have been ignored or concealed before being presented to the doctor.

Male 'breast swelling'

Swelling of the breast area in a man is nowadays commonly due to fatty tissue and is secondary to being overweight. In this case the swelling is equal on both sides, is soft, there are no distinct lumps or any abnormality of the skin or the nipple and the man will be obviously carrying too much weight anyway. This is not true breast swelling, but is just excess fat, which gives the appearance of breast enlargement.

True breast tissue enlargement in men is called gynaecomastia, and it is less common. Adolescent boys often show temporary gynaecomastia, which is normal and resolves spontaneously in all but a minority. Adult gynaecomastia can be caused as a side effect of several drugs, most notably some of those used to treat heart disorders, high blood pressure, stomach ulcers or prostate cancer. Other possible causes include rare hormone and genetic conditions. Gynaecomastia is also seen in long-term alcoholics. It will usually be easy for a GP to distinguish true gynaecomastia from excess fat but the advice of a specialist may be needed to determine the exact cause of the gynaecomastia.

Diagnosis

There should be no difficulty in distinguishing gynaecomastia, which is harmless although can cause cosmetic embarrassment, from breast cancer. In men the usual symptom of breast cancer is a lump or distortion of the overlying skin or the nipple on one side of the chest. The same techniques as are used in women, such as mammography, fine needle aspiration of cells and tissue biopsy can be used to confirm the diagnosis.

As with female breast cancer, lengthy delay in seeking medical advice about a lump can result in the cancer reaching a more advanced stage, and consequently becoming more difficult to treat. Awareness of male breast cancer is low, and men in general are not good at presenting themselves to doctors when they don't feel well or when they discover something wrong with them. Hopefully time and better availability of information will reduce the delay in detection of male breast cancer.

Treatment

This follows similar lines to female treatment. If the cancer is small enough to be removed as a lump plus a margin of normal tissue (wide local excision, WLE), then this will be done along with removal of axillary lymph nodes (possibly using the sentinel node biopsy technique first). A modified radical mastectomy (page 74) is however the commoner procedure needed in men, because there is less surrounding tissue to give a safe margin and also because of the tendency to be more locally advanced at the time of diagnosis. Radiotherapy thereafter is routine.

Adjuvant treatment is applied in a similar way to female breast cancer. The majority of male breast cancers are ER +ve, and so tamoxifen can be used. Chemotherapy is given for ER -ve cancers or when there has been spread to the lymph nodes or beyond.

Chapter 10

Preventing Breast Cancer

Much effort has been put into research on ways to prevent breast cancer occurring and the results are summarised in the next few pages. A brief search on the Internet or in a large bookstore will also reveal plenty of evidence of diets that are supposed to reduce breast cancer risk, or food supplements that do the same. It is entirely understandable that there should be such interest in 'natural' ways of reducing risk. Much of this self-help information is well-intentioned but some of it is misinformed or even exploitative. It's therefore useful to look at the extent of the scientific evidence that exists for breast cancer prevention.

Diet

FAT

Dietary fat is strongly suspected of being important in the cause of many cancers and the possibility of a link to breast cancer was mentioned in chapter 2. The concept of being able to reduce risk by a change in diet is of course very attractive, not least because it would offer a means of active resistance against disease that we could all take up.

A positive relationship between saturated fats (the types that are solid at room temperature and typically come from animal sources) has both been demonstrated and refuted. This confusing picture may largely be because of the difficulty in carrying out accurate dietary assessments in the population. We don't know for example if a person's diet in childhood is more or less important than it is in adulthood, and asking an adult to remember what their diet consisted of when they were young children could never be an exact exercise. People's diets change over the years, so it may be that there needs to be a certain factor in the diet over a minimum length of time before a change is seen, and so on. The best that can be currently said is that there is a *possible* link between saturated fat and breast cancer. Since we already know that increased levels of dietary saturated fat intake are associated with greater likelihood of developing heart and blood vessel disease this at least ties in with what we already know about what constitutes healthy eating.

There is no definite evidence that consuming a smaller amount of saturated fat in the diet will lead to less likelihood of developing breast cancer, and even less evidence in favour of a prolonged survival from breast cancer that might be attributable to diet, but there is enough general evidence to recommend such a diet in any case. There is certainly *no* evidence to suggest that a reduced fat diet of the 'healthy' variety we're here referring to causes any *increase* in breast cancer.

ISOFLAVONES

There is much current research interest in a group of food compounds called isoflavones, which are in turn part of a bigger group of compounds called phytoestrogens. Phytoestrogens are, literally, oestrogen-like substances and they have been found in over 300 types of plant. The two main subdivisions are known as lignans (present in flaxseed, linseed and wholegrain cereals) and isoflavones (present in pulses like soy beans and chick peas and in clovers). Soy is particularly high in phytoestrogens and was mentioned in chapter 2 as one of the possible protecting factors that accounts for the low incidence of breast cancer in Japanese women. Other foodstuffs in which these compounds are found include apples, carrots, coffee, potatoes, yams, bean sprouts, sunflower and sesame seeds, rye and wheat.

Laboratory work has indicated that isoflavones may reduce the tendency for breast tumours to develop, but this is a long way from being applicable to real life in human beings. Promensil is an extract of red clover containing isoflavones, which is currently under clinical trials. The results of such investigations are many years away.

ANTIOXIDANTS

The body constantly reacts with oxygen as part of the energy producing processes of cells. As a consequence of this activity, highly reactive molecules are produced known as free radicals. These interact with other molecules within the cell, which can cause oxidative damage to proteins, cell membranes and genes. This damage has been implicated in the cause of many diseases including cancers and has an impact on the body's aging process.

Antioxidants are substances that neutralise free radicals and the body produces an armoury of them to defend itself. The metabolic processes that produce antioxidants are controlled and influenced by an individual's genetic makeup and the extra environmental factors (such as diet, smoking and pollution) to which your body is exposed. Unfortunately, changes in our lifestyles that include more environmental pollution and less quality in our diets mean that we are exposed to more free radicals than ever before. Our internal production of antioxidants is insufficient to neutralize and scavenge all the free radicals but there is an abundant supply of antioxidants in a wide variety of foods. By increasing our dietary intake of antioxidants, we can help our body to defend itself. It's generally accepted that adequate amounts of antioxidants in the diet are protective against cancers in general and probably also have other health benefits. Although they have not specifically been shown to protect against breast cancer there is nonetheless enough evidence to indicate that diets high in antioxidants are desirable.

Examples of food-based antioxidants include:

- The vitamins (vitamin E, vitamin C, and beta carotene).
- The trace elements that are components of antioxidant enzymes (including selenium, copper, zinc, and manganese).
- Some non-nutrients such as ubiquinone (coenzyme Q) which is sometimes used as an 'energy booster'; phytoestrogens are themselves antioxidants.
- Lycopene, a pigment found in tomatoes and responsible for the red colour; it is also a powerful antioxidant. Tomatoes in all their forms are the major source of lycopene and include tomato products like canned tomatoes, tomato soup, tomato juice and even ketchup. Lycopene is also highly concentrated in watermelon.
- Beta-carotene, which is an orange pigment first isolated from carrots 150 years ago. It is found concentrated in deep orange and green vegetables (the green chlorophyll covers up the orange pigment). Carrots also contain phytoestrogens.

Oranges, grapefruit, lemons and limes possess many natural substances that appear to be important in disease protection. Together these 'phytochemicals' act more powerfully than if they were given separately. Black tea, green tea and oolong teas also have antioxidant properties. All three varieties come from the plant called *Camellia sinenis*. Common brands of black tea do contain antioxidants, but the most potent is green tea (jasmine tea), which contains the antioxidant catechin. Oolong tea has only 40 per cent as much of the antioxidants found in green tea and black tea has only 10 per cent as much. When green tea is processed (baked and fermented) to make black tea, some of the catechins are destroyed.

The evidence for dietary protection against breast cancer is therefore weak, although probably not absent. When it comes to looking at preventive measures that have the best scientific foundation then one has to concentrate on medications, particularly tamoxifen but also a small number of newer drugs.

Tamoxifen

Early clinical experience with the use of tamoxifen as adjuvant treatment in stage I and stage II breast cancer showed that it also reduced the likelihood of cancer developing in the opposite breast. This suggested a protective effect and several studies were then set up to investigate this further.

The National Surgical Adjuvant Breast and Bowel Project (NSABP) was an American study started in 1992 that was actually stopped early because those women receiving tamoxifen were only half as likely to develop breast cancer as those who did not receive tamoxifen. The early cessation of the trial made it impossible to conclude that the use of tamoxifen ultimately helped women to survive longer, because there were some disadvantages too. There was an increased chance of treated women developing clots in the veins and of getting cancer of the lining of the womb (endometrial carcinoma).

Early reports of the major international, UK-based trial also showed a benefit in breast cancer prevention for women who took tamoxifen. This was cancelled out by the side effects, including increased risk of other life-threatening conditions such as clots in the veins.

On balance current evidence suggests that the benefits of tamoxifen in breast cancer prevention *may* outweigh its risks in women who are:

- pre or post-menopausal but are at increased risk of developing breast cancer (see below for more detail on how this risk is estimated)
- post-menopausal and who have had their uterus removed (which means they cannot develop cancer of the womb)

Raloxifene

Tamoxifen is classed as a 'selective estrogen receptor modulator', or SERM. This means it blocks the action of oestrogen on some tissues (such as the breast) but not on others (such as the lining of the womb). Much research is currently underway to develop more specific SERM drugs that provide the benefits without the disadvantages, because we know that there are different types of oestrogen 'receptor' in different tissues.

Raloxifene is a SERM currently licensed in the UK to reduce the risk of a woman developing the weak bone condition called osteoporosis. Osteoporosis develops in post-menopausal women because oestrogen normally stimulates the bone-forming cells within the skeleton. After the menopause the natural drop in oestrogen causes an increased rate of bone loss, which can take years to slow down again. In the meantime much bone strength can be lost. Raloxifene partially prevents this from happening.

Several research studies have also suggested that raloxifene may reduce the likelihood of breast cancer occurring. Although raloxifene seems not to increase the chance of developing cancer of the lining of the womb it does increase the risk of blood clots in the veins. Other studies are presently in progress to define raloxifene's role more precisely, so at the moment it cannot be recommended as a defence against breast cancer.

Predicting the risk of breast cancer

Some of the studies into the role of drugs to protect against developing breast cancer have shown the best results only in women who are at above average risk. So the question of course arises, how can risk be assessed? Back in chapter 2, table 1, we listed some of the factors that can help to determine if a woman has a high genetic risk of developing breast cancer, but more sophisticated computerised 'calculators' have been developed. One well known one is the 'Gail' model, which takes into account various factors such as the age of first periods starting, age at first pregnancy, family history and so on. The result is presented as a score.

The Gail calculator is available for use on the Internet, and can be accessed on the web site of the National Cancer Institute (USA) at http://bcra.nci.nih.gov/brc/

Although many women will be interested to make use of such a calculator it's important to emphasise several points. First is that such tools are only meant as guides. It should be clear from the preceding chapters that we are ignorant of much important information concerning breast cancer, and we are unable to predict which women will and will not develop this disease. So the calculator is a rough guide only. It is best used in conjunction with your doctor or practice nurse and the results should form the basis for a discussion about breast health, not as a decision-making device in its own right. Secondly, and most importantly, the result of such a calculation makes no difference to the need to be 'breast aware' and to report any new findings or symptoms without delay to your doctor. All women are at some risk of developing breast cancer, no matter what a calculator may say.

To put the Gail model results into the context of what was mentioned earlier about research trials, those who showed the greatest benefit from taking tamoxifen were:

- pre-menopausal with a Gail risk factor greater than 1.66 per cent
- post-menopausal with a Gail risk factor greater than 3 per cent

Aromatase inhibitors

Aromatase inhibitor drugs such as anastrozole reduce the output of oestrogen by fatty tissues and have been mentioned as adjuvant treatments for breast cancer. Several research trials have shown very encouraging results with anastrozole as potentially being capable of reducing breast cancer occurrence. More information is needed and it will be several years yet before we can be sure of the role of this drug and others like it, and how it compares against drugs like tamoxifen. At the moment it cannot be recommended for protection and in any case it would only be suitable for older, postmenopausal women.

Non-steroidal anti-inflammatory drugs

NSAIDs, as they are more conveniently called, are very widely used painkillers and anti-inflammatory medicines. Ibuprofen is the best known and there are dozens of others. There is some research to suggest that women who take NSAIDs regularly may have a smaller risk of developing breast cancer. However, NSAIDs also have many potential side effects, among them ulcers and bleeding from the digestive system. There is no evidence to properly inform their use as protectors against breast cancer, so they cannot be recommended for that purpose.

Women at very high risk

A small number of women are at particularly high risk of developing breast cancer. Such women usually have a strongly positive family history of the disease and they may also be carriers of the 'breast cancer genes', BRCA1 and BRCA2. The risk of breast cancer can be as high as 50 per cent in women with these genes and they should be offered expert counselling on what choices they have with a specialist in genetics, as well as with the breast cancer team. Their options include intensive screening, possibly combined with anti-oestrogen drugs or surgery. Particularly in the USA, an increasing number of high-risk women are opting to have their breasts removed in order to reduce their risk as much as possible.

Such a dramatic step is never undertaken lightly, yet the results of 'prophylactic mastectomy' as it's called are far from clear. First, the risk of breast cancer is not reduced to zero. If small amounts of breast tissue remain then they can still turn cancerous, so the surgical skill and experience of the surgeon can have a direct bearing on the end result. Secondly, the relatively small total number of women who undergo this procedure, combined with the lack of an exactly comparable group of women who receive no protective treatment makes it very difficult to say for sure that removing the breasts results in a longer and healthier life. As with most such important issues there are heavy weights on both sides of the balance, and only careful individual assessment and discussion can help each woman make the decision that's best for her.

Conclusion

Breast cancer has proved to be one of the biggest modern health challenges, particularly for women in industrialised societies. It is getting commoner and it obeys its own rule book. It remains difficult to achieve predictable long-term cure in the same way as for many other cancers seen and treated well at an early stage, but the tide is on the turn. Knowledge is rapidly expanding and many very promising drugs are already showing excellent results. The full range of anti-cancer treatments can be brought to bear on breast cancer and we are getting better at combining them to achieve the best results with the least side effects. Proper attention too is being paid to the psychological consequences of breast cancer and the effects that the loss of a breast can have on a woman. Treatment for this aspect of the disease has advanced well. There is excellent support in the way of voluntary organisations and information services, details of which are in appendix C.

Breast cancer need not be feared. It will not happen to the majority of women and those women who are affected can count on the best of support and services in the UK.

Appendix A

References

- Early Breast Trialists' Collaborative Group, 'Systemic treatment of early breast cancer by hormonal, cytotoxic or immune therapy' (Lancet, 1992; 339: 1–15, 71–85); www.thelancet.com
- Early Breast Trialists' Collaborative Group, 'Tamoxifen for early breast cancer: an overview of the randomised trials' (Lancet, 1998; 351: 1451–67).
- Early Breast Trialists' Collaborative Group, 'Polychemotherapy for early breast cancer: an overview of the randomised trials' (Lancet, 1998; 352: 930–42).
- Cuzick, J., et al., 'Overview of the main outcomes in breast cancer prevention trials' (Lancet, 2003; 361: 296–300).
- Baum, M., 'The changing face of breast cancer – past, present and future perspectives' (Breast Cancer Research and Treatment, 2002; 75: S1–S5).

- Key, T. J., et al., 'The effect of diet on risk of cancer' (Lancet, 2002; 360: 861–68).
- Bingham, S., et al., 'Are imprecise methods obscuring a relation between fat and breast cancer?' (Lancet, 2003; 362: 212–14).
- Prichard, R. S., et al., 'The prevention of breast cancer' (British Journal of Surgery, 2003; 90: 772–83).
- Berg, J., 'Breast cancer prevention: is the risk-benefit ratio in favour of tamoxifen?' (Lancet, 2003; 362: 183–84).
- Beral, V., et al., 'Breast cancer and hormone replacement therapy in the Million Women Study' (Lancet, 2003; 362: 419–27).
- Cann, S. A., et al., 'Hypothesis: iodine, selenium and the development of breast cancer' (Cancer Causes & Control, 2000; 11(2): 121–27).
- Sakorafas, G. H., 'The management of women at high risk for the development of breast cancer: risk estimation and preventative strategies' (Cancer Treatment Reviews, 2003; 29: 79–89).
- Perkins, G. H., and Middleton, L. P., 'Breast cancer in men' (British Medical Journal, 2003; 327: 239–40); http://bmj.com/cgi/content/full/327/7409/239.
- British Medical Journal: collected resources on breast cancer: http://bmj.com/cgi/collection/cancer%3Abreast
- National Institute for Clinical Excellence, 'Breast cancer service guidance'; http://www.nice.org.uk/cat.asp?c=36017 (other guidelines on the use of specific breast cancer drugs can be found by searching the NICE site using the drug name).
- Dixon, M. J. (editor), 'ABC of Breast Diseases', 2nd edition, BMJ Books (2000).

Appendix B

Drugs

The following information contains selected details of some of the medications used in treating breast cancer. Full details are included in the manufacturers' data sheets and can also be viewed within the medicines section of the NetDoctor web site http://www.netdoctor.co.uk/medicines/

The information is accurate at the time of writing but new information on medicines appears regularly. A health professional should always be consulted concerning the prescription and use of medicines.

Medicines and their possible side effects can affect individual people in different ways. The following lists some of the side effects that are known to be associated with these medicines. Side effects other than those listed may exist.

Selective estrogen receptor modulators (SERM)

TAMOXIFEN

This medicine contains the active ingredient tamoxifen citrate, which is a type of medicine known as an 'anti-oestrogen'. It is mainly used to treat women with breast cancers that respond to the female sex hormone, oestrogen. Most breast cancers are sensitive to oestrogen, and their growth is increased in the presence of this hormone. Oestrogen binds to oestrogen receptors on the breast cancer cells and causes changes within the cells that result in faster growth of the cancer. Tamoxifen works by blocking these oestrogen receptors, thereby blocking the effect of oestrogen on the cancer. This reduces the size of oestrogen-sensitive tumours.

Cautions

As this medicine may potentially cause harm to a developing baby, it should not be used during pregnancy. Pre-menopausal women should use a non-hormonal method of contraception to prevent pregnancy both during, and for two months following, treatment with this medicine.

Tamoxifen is associated with a small increase in the risk of endometrial cancer. The benefits of taking tamoxifen to treat breast cancer outweigh this risk. However, to minimise the risk you should consult your doctor if you experience any abnormal gynaecological symptoms during or after treatment, so that they can be investigated. Symptoms to report include vaginal bleeding, menstrual irregularities, vaginal discharge, or symptoms such as pelvic pain or pressure. Consult your doctor for further information.

Tamoxifen is associated with an increased risk of abnormal blood clots in the blood vessels (deep vein thrombosis or pulmonary embolism), particularly during periods of immobilisation and following surgery. The benefits of taking tamoxifen to treat breast cancer outweigh this risk. However, you should consult your doctor immediately if you experience any of the following symptoms during treatment: stabbing pains and/or unusual swelling in one leg, pain on breathing or coughing, sudden breathlessness or sudden severe chest pain. Consult your doctor for further information.

Main side effects
- headache
- blood disorders
- disturbances of the gut such as diarrhoea, constipation, nausea, vomiting or abdominal pain
- visual disturbances
- severe swelling of lips, face or tongue (angioedema)
- the presence of tissue similar to the lining of the uterus at other sites in the pelvis (endometriosis)
- severe blistering skin reaction affecting the tissues of the eyes, mouth, throat and genitals (Stevens-Johnson Syndrome)
- suppression of menstrual periods
- stimulation of tumour growth
- hair loss
- liver disorders
- itching of the external female genitalia
- cancerous changes in the endometrium (lining of the womb)
- increased risk of abnormal blood clots within the blood vessels
- fibroids in the womb (uterus)
- vaginal bleeding or discharge
- hot flushes

How can this medicine affect other medicines?
Tamoxifen increases the anti-blood-clotting effects of the anticoagulant medicines nicoumalone and warfarin. Women taking anticoagulants in combination with tamoxifen should have their blood-clotting times

regularly monitored, and your doctor may need to reduce the dose of your anticoagulant. There may be an increased risk of abnormal blood clots in the veins (thromboembolism) if tamoxifen is taken with cytotoxic chemotherapy medicines.

RALOXIFENE

Raloxifene is a selective estrogen receptor modulator (SERM). It has actions similar to those of oestrogen on bone tissue, but not on uterine or breast tissues.

At the menopause blood levels of oestrogen (the main female sex hormone) decrease, which leads to a loss of bone density. Bone loss is particularly rapid for the first ten years after the menopause. This may lead to the development of osteoporosis – a condition in which the bones are brittle and break more easily. Raloxifene binds to oestrogen receptors and stimulates their action in bone and the cardiovascular system. This leads to an eventual increase in the density of bone. Raloxifene is used to treat post-menopausal osteoporosis. It is not useful in the treatment of menopausal symptoms such as hot flushes. Raloxifene has also been shown to reduce the incidence of breast cancer in women taking it for protection against osteoporosis.

Main side effects
- swelling of the legs and ankles due to excess fluid retention (peripheral oedema)
- leg cramps
- hot flushes
- blood clots in the veins

How can this medicine affect other medicines?
The absorption of raloxifene is reduced by cholestyramine and it is recommended that they are not used together.

When used together with warfarin or nicoumalone, raloxifene may reduce the blood thinning effects of these medicines.

Chemotherapy

PACLITAXEL

Paclitaxel is an anti-cancer medicine known as a 'taxane'. Cancers form when some cells within the body multiply uncontrollably and abnormally. These cells then spread and invade nearby tissues. Paclitaxel works by stopping the cancer cells from dividing and multiplying. This kills the cancer cells and stops the cancer growing.

Unfortunately, paclitaxel also affects normal, healthy cells, particularly those that multiply quickly such as blood cells. The most important side effect is on the bone marrow where blood cells are made. Paclitaxel can decrease the production of blood cells, leaving people susceptible to infection. Regular blood tests are therefore needed to monitor levels of blood cells.

Paclitaxel is usually given in hospital as a three-hour infusion into a vein (intravenously), with a three-week interval between treatment courses. A corticosteroid, an antihistamine and an H2 antagonist such as cimetidine or ranitidine will also be prescribed before the infusion. This is to reduce the chance of experiencing allergic reactions to the medicine or the severity of any reactions. The aim of the treatment is to progressively shrink the cancer over several cycles of chemotherapy, allowing normal, healthy cells to recover in between.

Paclitaxel is licensed to treat cancer of the ovaries (ovarian cancer), breast cancer and lung cancer.

Main side effects

- diarrhoea
- low blood pressure (hypotension)
- hair loss (alopecia)
- decreased production of blood cells by the bone marrow (bone marrow suppression)
- increased susceptibility to infections
- disorder of the peripheral nerves causing weakness and numbness (peripheral neuropathy)
- nausea and vomiting
- low red blood cell count (anaemia)
- slow heart rate (bradycardia)
- pain and swelling at site of injection
- allergy to active ingredients (hypersensitivity) such as facial flushing, skin rash, itch, narrowing of airways (bronchospasm) or swelling of lips, tongue or throat (angioedema)
- pain in the muscles and joints
- inflamed and sore mouth

How can this medicine affect other medicines?

Chemotherapy decreases the body's immune response. This means that vaccines may be less effective if given during treatment, and live vaccines may cause serious infections. Live vaccines include: measles, mumps, rubella, MMR, oral polio, oral typhoid and yellow fever.

CYCLOPHOSPHAMIDE

Cyclophosphamide is one of a group of anti-cancer medicines called 'alkylating agents'. Apart from breast cancer it is also used in the treatment of a wide variety of other cancers including of the lymph nodes (lymphoma) and blood cells (leukaemias). It is usually used in combination with other anti-cancer medicines.

Cyclophosphamide can be taken either by mouth as tablets or by slow infusion into the veins (intravenously). In some cases a medicine called Mesna (Uromitexan) is also given to reduce the adverse effects of cyclophosphamide on the bladder (urinary tract). Drinking plenty of fluids when taking cyclophosphamide also helps to reduce the severity of bladder irritation.

Main side effects
- decreased production of blood cells by the bone marrow (bone marrow suppression)
- retention of water in the body tissues (fluid retention), resulting in swelling (oedema)
- dizziness
- nausea and vomiting
- inflammation of the bladder causing bleeding (haemorrhagic cystitis)
- low blood sodium level (hyponatraemia)
- hair loss (alopecia) with long-term use of medication

DOXORUBICIN
Doxorubicin belongs to a group of anti-cancer medicines called cytotoxic anthracycline antibiotics. These are synthetic medicines that have been derived from compounds found in certain bacteria and fungi. Doxorubicin's exact mechanism of action is unknown but it seems to work in three ways. It inserts itself into the strands of genetic material (DNA) inside the cell and binds them together. This prevents the cell from making genetic material (DNA and RNA) and proteins. It also appears to interfere with an enzyme called topoisomerase II, which is involved in DNA replication. Finally it can also form free radicals, which are molecules capable of damaging cells. All this prevents the cell from growing and therefore it dies. As with all anti-cancer drugs the growth and division of normal, healthy cells is also affected.

Main side effects

- rash
- disturbances of the gut such as diarrhoea, constipation, nausea, vomiting or abdominal pain
- allergic reaction to the active ingredient
- hair loss (alopecia)
- fever
- low red blood cell count (anaemia)
- loss of appetite
- decrease in the number of white blood cells in the blood (leucopenia)
- inflammation of the lining of the mouth (stomatitis)
- damage to the heart (cardiotoxicity)
- weakness or loss of strength (asthenia)
- decrease in the number of platelets in the blood (thrombocytopenia)
- painful redness, swelling, blistering or ulceration of the palms and soles

FLUOROURACIL (5-FLUOROURACIL)

Fluorouracil is one of a group of anti-cancer medicines called 'cytotoxic antimetabolites'. It can be given by mouth either as capsules or the solution can be mixed in with fruit juice. It can also be given by injection or slow infusion into the veins (intravenously).

Main side effects

- diarrhoea
- visual disturbances
- nausea and vomiting
- skin darkening
- decrease in the number of white blood cells in the blood (leucopenia)
- hair loss (alopecia)
- chest pain

- decreased production of blood cells by the bone marrow (bone marrow suppression)

METHOTREXATE

Methotrexate is a type of medicine called a cytotoxic antimetabolite. It is used to treat three different conditions: rheumatoid arthritis, psoriasis and cancer of various types.

Methotrexate works by inhibiting the action of an enzyme called dihydrofolate reductase. This enzyme normally converts folic acid into a substance called tetrahydrofolic acid, which is essential for the synthesis of new genetic material (DNA) within cells. Cells are unable to divide, multiply and repair themselves without tetrahydrofolic acid to make new DNA. As methotrexate deprives cells of this nutrient it kills cancer cells and stops the cancer growing.

Unfortunately, methotrexate also affects the division of normal, healthy cells, particularly those that divide rapidly such as the cells lining the mouth and gut and cells in the bone marrow. For this reason, cancer chemotherapy using high doses of methotrexate is usually followed by a treatment called folinic acid rescue therapy. This involves giving tetrahydrofolic acid, in the form of folinic acid (also called calcium folinate or calcium leucovorin), usually 24 hours after the methotrexate. This bypasses the action of the methotrexate and allows normal cell division to recover. Normal healthy cells recover faster than cancer cells and this helps to prevent side effects. The aim is to progressively shrink the cancer over several cycles of chemotherapy, allowing normal cells to recover in between.

Methotrexate is used to treat a wide variety of cancers, including acute leukaemias, non-Hodgkin's lymphoma, soft tissue and bone cancers, and solid tumours, particularly breast, lung, head and neck, bladder, cervical, ovarian, and testicular cancers. It may be given by mouth or injection, depending on the dose, and is most commonly used in combination with other chemotherapy medicines.

Methotrexate is used in lower doses taken by mouth to treat severe rheumatoid arthritis and severe psoriasis that have not responded to other treatments.

Main side effects
- headache
- blurred vision
- diarrhoea
- changes in mood
- drowsiness
- fatigue
- lung disorders
- abnormal reaction of the skin to light, usually a rash (photo-sensitivity)
- hair loss (alopecia)
- nausea and vomiting
- low red blood cell count (anaemia)
- decrease in the number of white blood cells in the blood (leucopenia)
- inflammation of the lining of the mouth (stomatitis)
- shaky movements and unsteady walk (ataxia)
- irritation of the eye
- decrease in the number of platelets in the blood (thrombocytopenia)
- liver disorders
- a general feeling of being unwell
- ulceration or bleeding of the stomach or intestines
- rash or itching
- kidney disorders
- decrease in fertility (reversible on stopping treatment)

How can this medicine affect other medicines?

The following medicines must not be taken by people receiving methotrexate:

- co-trimoxazole (antibiotic)
- trimethoprim (antibiotic)
- nitrous oxide (anaesthetic)

Salicylate medicines such as aspirin, and non-steroidal anti-inflammatory drugs (NSAIDs) such as ibuprofen, ketoprofen and diclofenac can reduce the removal of methotrexate from the body. This can cause levels of methotrexate to build up in the blood, increasing the risk of side effects. For this reason, people taking methotrexate should avoid buying aspirin or NSAIDs such as ibuprofen to take as painkillers or anti-inflammatories. These medicines should only be used on the advice of the doctor who is monitoring your methotrexate treatment, so that changes can be made to your methotrexate dose if necessary. Check with your doctor before taking vitamin preparations that contain folic acid.

Vaccines may be less effective in people taking this medicine. This is because methotrexate reduces the activity of the immune system and can prevent the body forming adequate antibodies. Live vaccines should be avoided where possible because they may cause infection. Live vaccines include the following: oral polio; rubella; measles, mumps and rubella (MMR); BCG; yellow fever and oral typhoid vaccines.

TRASTUZUMAB

Trastuzumab is a type of medicine called a humanised monoclonal antibody. Monoclonal antibodies are proteins that are synthetically designed to recognise other proteins called antigens.

Trastuzumab is used to treat tumours that have large amounts of a unique antigen called human epidermal growth factor receptor 2 protein (HER2) on the surface of the cancer cells. HER2 is present in excessive amounts on the surface of some breast cancer cells, and its presence stimulates the growth of these cancer cells.

Trastuzumab works by recognising HER2 on the surface of cancer cells. It binds to HER2 and by doing so, inhibits its function. This stops the growth of the cancer cells.

Trastuzumab is used to treat breast cancer that has large amounts of HER2 on its cells, and has spread to other areas of the body. It is used on its own when at least two other chemotherapy treatments have proved unsuccessful, and can also be used in combination with the chemotherapy agent paclitaxel, as first line treatment.

Main side effects
- headache
- rash
- inability of the heart to pump blood efficiently (heart failure)
- depression
- difficulties with breathing
- blood disorders
- disturbances of the gut such as diarrhoea, constipation, nausea, vomiting or abdominal pain
- lung disorders
- fever (pyrexia)
- chills
- pins and needles (paraesthesia)
- dizziness
- excessive fluid retention in the body tissues, resulting in swelling (oedema)
- chest pain
- increased heart rate (tachycardia)

- anxiety
- pain in the muscles and joints
- liver or kidney disorders

VINORELBINE

Vinorelbine belongs to a group of anti-cancer medicines called vinca alkaloids. Alkaloids prevent the chromosomes within the nucleus of cells, and which contain the genetic information, forming the spindles necessary for cell duplication. Vinorelbine is used principally in combination with other anticancer medicines and is administered by intravenous injection or infusion only.

Main side effects
- constipation
- pins and needles (paraesthesia)
- nausea and vomiting
- low red blood cell count (anaemia)
- pain at injection site
- inflammation of the wall of a vein (phlebitis)
- reversible hair loss
- decrease in the number of a type of white blood cell (neutrophil) in the blood (neutropenia)
- jaw pain
- decrease in the number of platelets in the blood (thrombocytopenia)
- disorder of the peripheral nerves causing weakness and numbness (peripheral neuropathy)

Drugs sometimes used in the treatment of breast pain (mastalgia)

DANAZOL

Danazol structurally resembles a group of natural hormones (androgens) found in the body. It acts on part of the brain called the pituitary gland, which produces a range of hormones that control various aspects of the body's metabolism. Danazol specifically decreases the production of those hormones that are responsible for menstruation and ovulation. Apart from mastalgia it is also used to treat abnormal menstrual bleeding.

Main side effects

- blurred vision
- muscle cramps
- blood disorders
- hair loss (alopecia)
- flushing
- increased hair growth (hirsutism)
- vaginal dryness
- disorders of the menstrual cycle
- weight gain
- acne
- voice changes
- reduced breast size in women

BROMOCRIPTINE

Bromocriptine works by stimulating dopamine receptors in the brain. This has several results and hence its several uses. Stimulating dopamine receptors causes a decrease in the production of the hormone prolactin from the pituitary gland in the brain. High prolactin levels are associated with many conditions including some breast disorders and tumours of the pituitary gland. Reducing prolactin levels therefore improves symptoms of these conditions.

Main side effects
- headache
- constipation
- dry mouth
- drowsiness
- difficulty performing voluntary movements, resulting in jerky or involuntary movements or muscle twitches (dyskinesia)
- dizziness
- nausea and vomiting

How can this medicine affect other medicines?
Alcohol may increase adverse effects of bromocriptine. If this occurs, the use of alcohol should be stopped for the duration of this treatment.

Some antibiotics from the group called the macrolides (e.g. erythromycin) may increase the levels of bromocriptine in the body. Individuals taking this combination must be monitored.

Appendix C

Useful Contacts

Breast cancer care

www.breastcancercare.org.uk
Breast Cancer Care is the leading provider of breast cancer information
and support across the UK. Services are free and include a help line,
web site, publications, and practical and emotional support.

Regional offices:
61–63 St John Street
London EC1M 4AN
Tel: 020 7566 5880

North & Midlands Regional Centre
19 Paradise Square
Sheffield S1 1JG
Tel: 0114 276 0296

Floor 4
40 St Enoch Square
Glasgow G1 4DH
Tel: 0141 221 2244

First Floor
14 Cathedral Road
Cardiff CF11 9LJ
Tel: 029 2023 4070

Breakthrough Breast Cancer

www.breakthrough.org.uk
Breakthrough Breast Cancer is a charity committed to fighting breast
cancer through research and awareness.

Breakthrough Breast Cancer
3rd Floor Kingsway House
103 Kingsway
London WC2B 6QX
Tel: 020 7405 5111

CancerHelp UK

www.cancerhelp.org.uk
www.cancer.org.uk
CancerHelp UK is a free information service about cancer and cancer care for people with cancer and their families. It is the public information arm of Cancer Research UK, the largest volunteer-supported cancer research organisation in the world.

Macmillan Cancer Relief

www.macmillan.org.uk
Macmillan Cancer Relief is a UK charity that works to improve the quality of life for people living with cancer. Macmillan offers the expert care and practical support that makes a difference to people living with cancer.

Macmillan Cancer Line (Mon–Fri 9 a.m.–6 p.m.): 0808 8082020

Maggie's Centres

www.maggiescentres.org
The aim of Maggie's Centres is to help people with cancer to be as healthy in mind and body as possible and enable them to make their own contribution to their medical treatment and recovery.

They are also for their families, their friends and their carers. If they want to, they can share their experiences with others in similar situations and, with professional help, inform themselves about the medical realities of their disease. Each centre is close to a major cancer hospital treatment centre.